Creating and Maintaining Balance

A WOMAN'S GUIDE TO SAFE, NATURAL HORMONE HEALTH

By Holly Lucille, ND, RN

Foreword By Jacob Teitelbaum, MD

IMPAKT|health

Published by:
IMPAKT Health
2551 31st St.
Boulder, CO 80301
E-mail: info@impakt.com
Fax: 303-440-7446
www.impakt.com

Publishers' note:

The information herein can be a valuable addition to your doctor's
advice, but it is not intended to replace the services of a trained professional.
It is not safe to self-diagnose. If you have symptoms suggestive of a condition discussed in this book, please consult a healthcare practitioner,
preferably a naturopathic doctor (ND).

Before experimenting with natural treatments, discuss them with your
care provider. Since many conventional healthcare practitioners may not be
aware of the natural alternatives available, you may need to help educate
him or her. Bring this book along with you to the doctor's office.

DEDICATION

This book is for all women looking for a safe, natural, effective way to deal with hormone health in our modern times. I am fully aware that there are many options to choose from when it comes to taking care of oneself. No matter what choices we make to remedy what ails us, there are two ingredients that cannot be left out, or any attempt will be useless. Those ingredients are love and compassion. I would like to give special thanks to the women in my life who have taught me most about these aspects of myself:

Lucille Niebel,

Naomi,

and Cathy.

TABLE OF CONENTS

Acknowledgments

It takes us all to make the world go around, and nearly as many people to create a project like this. It has been a wonderful honor to work with so many extraordinary people, and I would like to thank you all.

Thanks to everyone at Enzymatic Therapy for continuing to help people know what better feels like.

To Miriam Weidner and Linda Knittel at IMPAKT Health, you are simply brilliant. Karolyn Gazella, your gifts and patience are invaluable. Dena Nishek, what a beautiful blessing you are—thank you for your care, gifts, and gentleness.

To my friends and family who make me who I am. And thanks to my patients, with whom I am privileged to work and without whom I am nothing.

BY JACOB TEITELBAUM, MD

Foreword

Medicine is evolving. When I was in medical school in the early 1970s, the focus of treatment was how to "poison" one body system to remedy another. A contemporary example is Prozac, which poisons the system that brings serotonin into cells for storage, thus raising extracellular serotonin levels. This can work well to treat depression, but altering one system often throws others out of balance. For example, Prozac also causes sexual dysfunction and other side effects in approximately one-third of the people who use it. Nonetheless, in a society based on economics and quick fixes, prescription medications and surgery have surged ahead of other healing arts. Although there are certain benefits to this approach, there are also great costs for patients.

By learning how healthcare came to be the way it is today, we gain understanding and the ability to choose where we want to go. In the 1800s, there was little research and regulation in the healing arts. For much of human history, treatments were based on hundreds or thousands of years of experience and social traditions. The healers and wise women in the tribe would learn what worked from experience and pass on the information to their apprentices in a chain that often spanned thousands of years. As world wars and the expansion of Western civilization began to destroy long-standing social structures around the planet, much of this information and experience was lost. Accountability was also lost, and we began to see the rise of snake oil salesmen—people selling so-called natural remedies that actually had no health benefits. Natural medicine entered a period of decline.

It was in this context that science came to the forefront. People longed for proven healthcare methods developed by people who were accountable for their claims. Scientists provided this, using techniques that allowed ideas to be tested, reproduced, and validated. Because of the natural competition in the field, these ideas initially had to survive other scientists' skepticism before being accepted. Testing and validation began to take hold in the healing arts.

As in any system that generates a large amount of money and power, factors other than truth began to have their say. In the early 1900s, research focused on both biophysics (treatments that affect the body's energy systems) and biochemistry (treatments that modify chemical reactions in the body). Because the biochemists had more money and political clout than the biophysicists, they gained the upper hand. *Who* you know can be more powerful than *what* you know, and the rise of biochemistry over biophysics had little to do with how effective and safe a treatment was. The lower standing of biophysicists meant research and treatment using biophysics was marginalized and suppressed. Seeing which way the winds of change were blowing, many of the greatest names in modern medicine switched from biophysics to biochemistry.

Medical schools were founded (many of which initially focused on using natural therapies), standardized curricula and tests were developed, and it became possible to develop reliable conditions for being licensed. To counteract snake oil salesmen who were preying on the public, state governments developed licensing requirements for the practice of the healing arts, bringing more credibility, power, and respect to the field. Medicine was therefore able to attract compassionate healers. The fields of allopathic medicine and chemistry flourished.

As our understanding of chemistry evolved, it began to change the face of our country. New chemically derived fibers and materials became a part of everyday living. We went from almost no foreign chemicals in our environment to thousands of new ones for our bodies to detoxify. These chemicals are part of our food and water supply, building materials, clothing, and—not surprisingly—our medications. Money fueled this development: A natural substance cannot be patented, but new chemicals can be. A patent prevents competition, so more money can be made. For example, to treat indigestion, patentable acid blockers can cost two dollars or more per pill, whereas nonpatentable calcium carbonate may cost a nickel. People realized there was a lot of money to be made in medicine and, in particular, patentable medications. Corporations used this money to influence legislation and people's perceptions in an attempt to eliminate competition.

Language was added to legislation to consolidate allopathic medicine's power. As the U.S. Food and Drug Administration (FDA) was developed to protect public safety in the face of thousands of new chemical treatments, language was also added to legislation stating manufacturers could not claim something was effective for treating an illness unless it went through the FDA approval process. This process costs $400 million to $800 million per treatment, so only treatments that can be patented (meaning not natural supplements) can recoup these enormous costs. An excellent example of the challenge faced by natural product manufacturers is the use of vitamin B6 for carpal tunnel syndrome. Treating carpal tunnel syndrome with 250 mg of B6 daily for six weeks costs about $9 per patient. Because the treatment cost is so low, vitamin B6 manufacturers would find it impossible to recoup the cost of getting FDA approval for this treatment. Without FDA approval, they cannot advertise B6 for this use. As such, most patients instead spend between $2,000 and $4,000 on surgery. The situation is the same for hundreds of other nonpatentable, effective, inexpensive, and relatively safe treatments. The FDA has even been fighting to prevent stores that sell supplements from handing out copies of scientific studies about supplements.

In one legislative stroke, it became illegal for the manufacturers of natural medicines and products to advertise or even give consumers information about how to treat illnesses, regardless of how good the scientific data supporting the claim. Legislation was also pushed through Congress allowing only medical doctors and osteopathic physicians to diagnose and treat people. It became illegal for other healthcare providers to give patients the information needed to make informed decisions. At the same time, medical schools taught students that nutritional and natural therapies had no scientific basis and were only used by quacks. Thus, despite a large body of scientific data supporting natural medicine, you may find your doctor uninformed about it, hostile to it, and resistant to even look at the studies. Modern medicine went from being the wonderful tool of science to becoming an exclusive belief system that rejects outside ideas.

Fortunately, as always, life moves forward seeking balance and growth. Although it has its strengths, allopathic medicine's weaknesses are becoming apparent. Despite lack of funding and acceptance by mainstream journals, research continues on natural and energy therapies (acupuncture, for example). Many practitioners are exploring this expanding body of research, but the majority in Western medicine has been hostile to this research and has turned a blind eye to it. So most medical doctors, like myself, often are introduced to this information by our patients.

As a physician, I was given the impression that if an important treatment existed for an illness, I had been taught about it. If someone claimed he or she could effectively treat a nontreatable disease, that person was a quack. If such a treatment existed, I would surely know about it.

I was wrong.

When I first started my practice, patients would ask me if I knew about certain herbal or nutritional treatments for illnesses. One patient asked me if I had ever heard about using coenzyme Q10 for congestive heart failure. "That's nonsense," I answered. "If coenzyme Q10 helped congestive heart failure, don't you think I would have been taught to use that instead of doing heart transplants?" Still, I said that I would look into it.

Joyce Miller, the librarian at Anne Arundel Medical Center in Annapolis, Md., has always been happy to procure studies for me (and she has gotten me many thousands through the years). When she did a literature search on coenzyme Q10, she found a number of studies showing it could be quite beneficial in treating congestive heart failure. I found this curious. During the following few months, this scene played out again and again. I decided to keep notes on these rare "pearls" in a 30-page spiral notebook. My notes are now more than a thousand pages long.

The area of natural medicine has been growing tremendously during the past few decades and can now treat many difficult and often debilitating conditions. For example, combining natural and prescription therapies has allowed us to develop highly effective treatments for people with chronic fatigue syndrome and fibromyalgia. These syndromes are characterized by exhaustion, widespread pain, "brain fog," and insomnia. They debilitate more than 6 million Americans. Most doctors tell their patients nothing can be done for these illnesses and the symptoms simply must be tolerated. Natural practitioners, however, know this is not the case. Well-conducted research demonstrates that more than 91 percent of patients can now find marked improvement using an integrative medical approach. In fact, natural medicine is now able to significantly improve the treatment of most illnesses.

So how can you get access to this information? Recognize that more than 95 percent of the clinical training your physician received was in treating severe, life-threatening illnesses. I was taught more about how to tell whether fluid coming from a patient's nose was from a skull fracture than I was taught about how to treat a common cold. It was somehow presumed that if a physician could save a person in a life-threatening emergency, he or she also would know how to treat common, nonemergency problems. As most of you with pain, fatigue, hormonal, or other day-to-day problems have learned, this is not the case.

A change is occurring in healthcare education, perhaps in response to the shortcomings of allopathic medicine. Schools of naturopathy have developed standardized, four-year curriculums and board exams that ensure excellent training and quality control. Naturopathic doctors are predominantly trained in treating day-to-day illness and in maintaining health—often with a mix of both natural and prescription therapies. I would certainly want to be treated with allopathic therapies in emergency situations such as a cardiac arrest or acute appendicitis, but naturopathic approaches can be powerful for treating day-to-day problems and maintaining optimum health.

Because of their training and the large body of scientific literature they are taught, naturopaths are being licensed as doctors by many states. In California, Holly Lucille, ND, RN, the author of this book, spearheaded this licensing. As president of the California Naturopathic Association, she is dedicated to making optimum health and healing available to everyone. Instead of poisoning your body with medications in an attempt to make you well, Dr. Lucille will teach you how to give your body what it needs to restore health and balance naturally. Although this approach may take a little longer—it takes longer to build a building than to tear one down—I think you'll find it feels much better than the healthcare you might be used to, and it is highly effective.

Dr. Lucille is passionate about giving people the information they need to restore and maintain optimum health safely. She is both incredibly knowledgeable and compassionate; I am honored to count her as a friend. This book is a breath of fresh air—I think you'll really enjoy it.

Love and best wishes,
Jacob Teitelbaum, MD

Dr. Teitelbaum is a board-certified internist and director of the Annapolis Research Center for Effective CFS/Fibromyalgia Therapies. Having suffered with and overcome these illnesses in 1975, he spent the next 25 years creating, researching, and teaching about effective therapies. He is the senior author of the landmark study *"Effective treatment of chronic fatigue syndrome and fibromyalgia—a placebo-controlled study"* (J Chronic Fatigue Syndr 18, 2001, 3-28; full text available at www.vitality101.com). *He lectures internationally and is author of the best-selling book* From Fatigued to Fantastic! *(Avery Penguin Putnam, 1996) and* Three Steps to Happiness! Healing Through Joy *(Deva Press, 2003).*

Introduction

Growing up the daughter of two pharmacists, I was well versed in the Western medical approach: "You don't feel well? Here take this pill." Even at a very young age, I had difficulties with this approach to health. I always wanted to know, "Why?" I wouldn't stop asking questions until things made sense to me. "What will it do for me? Will it hurt me? Will I need it all the time? How much does it cost?" My parents say I drove them crazy, leading them to hypothesize they had taken the wrong baby home from the hospital. However, my ability to question and the desire to know more has not stopped; in fact, it is why I'm writing this book about women's health. Fueled by curiosity and the desire to make a difference, I've learned women's health is much more than symptom management. It is about creating a balance in our exquisite collection of hormones through healthy living.

My professional journey began more than a decade ago when I decided to become a nurse because I wanted to help people. The inspiration came during a class for volunteers at a local hospital. I learned when people become ill or need to be hospitalized, they give up some of their personal rights, such as the right to privacy, the right to choose, and the right to be informed and understand all of what's going on. I was incensed and thought, "I have to get into this system and help."

But the questions didn't subside when I became a nurse. Soon, I was disillusioned with the simple directive of carrying out doctors' orders. I wanted more rationale behind some of the decisions being made. I wanted a more active role in caring for people.

In my quest to find a satisfying place for myself in healthcare, I found the American Holistic Nursing Association. Completing a post-graduate program in holistic nursing provided me with an environment in which I was guided by instruction and philosophy that supported and treated people, not just their diagnoses or symptoms. This felt perfect! After seven years in holistic nursing, becoming a naturopathic physician seemed the next natural step.

NATUROPATHIC THEORY

As a naturopathic doctor, I was taught to think about health and approach healing in a comprehensive—or holistic—way. Not only are naturopathic doctors trained in the medical and clinical sciences (biochemistry, pathophysiology, anatomy, and microbiology), we also are guided by principles and a unique philosophy of care. I use these principles to guide my practice.

• *First, do no harm*
Naturopathic doctors use methods and medicinal substances that minimize the risk of harmful side effects. They use interventions that exert the least possible force to restore health. They respect and work with each patient's inherent self-healing processes.

• *Identify and treat the cause*
The theory behind naturopathic medicine is to discover and then remove the underlying cause of an illness, not just eliminate or suppress symptoms. It is about restoring function in an individual, not artificially replacing it. Understanding symptom management and helping make people comfortable are extremely important; however, getting to the root of the problem is the goal.

• *Treat the whole person*
In naturopathic medicine, doctors recognize that people are more than just their physical bodies. People are complex beings bombarded by physical, mental, emotional, social, spiritual, biological, environmental, vocational, and many other influences that all contribute to their health and well-being. Naturopathic doctors look at all potential factors that might be contributing to a physical illness.

• *Doctor as teacher*
The Latin word for *doctor* also means *teacher*. Naturopathic doctors strive to educate their patients and work with them to optimize each patient's health. When people are informed, they are empowered. Educated people can take back responsibility for their health and their bodies.

- *Prevention is the cure*

Naturopathic medical theory is based on prevention. Each patient is treated as an individual, and his or her current and past health history is evaluated. Risk factors, including heredity and susceptibility to diseases, are explored; appropriate interventions are suggested to prevent illness. Paying attention to physical, emotional, and mental health throughout life can help prevent serious illness.

- *Nature's healing power*

Naturopathic doctors recognize that everyone has an inherent self-healing process that is ordered and intelligent. In practice, naturopaths support, facilitate, and assist this process by identifying and removing obstacles to health or correcting important deficiencies to create healthy internal and external environments.

As my private naturopathic practice evolved, I realized instead of a general family practice, I would be specializing in women's health. Day after day, appointment after appointment, women came to me for hormone-related issues. I saw women having difficulty transitioning into menopause, and I also saw an extraordinary number of younger women experiencing weight gain, irritability, insomnia, decreased libido, and hot flashes. There were also women with sexual and reproductive problems—infertility, uterine fibroids, endometriosis, ovarian cysts, and severe premenstrual syndrome (PMS)—as well as breast and uterine cancer. Most of these women came in with a recommendation from their physician that they begin taking synthetic hormones. For women entering menopause it was hormone replacement therapy (HRT), and for the younger women it was the birth control pill. In conventional medicine, the theory is that if declining hormones trigger menopausal symptoms, women should take "replacement" hormones to alleviate those symptoms. To treat PMS and other complaints, conventional medical doctors frequently prescribe birth control pills, which manipulate the body by providing replacement hormones throughout the month to moderate the effects of the natural hormone cycle. These artificial hormones suppress the body's natural cycle; they do nothing to address why the symptoms are occurring. Intuitively, these women knew synthetic hormones weren't the best solutions for them, so they came to me searching for something more.

A pattern was emerging among my patients, but it really hit home when my own 38-year-old body started to flare up. My periods became unbearable; I had cramping, clotting, and bloating. My PMS and irritability got so bad my family would mark the two weeks beforehand as the "red zone." I wrestled with debilitating fatigue for the first time in my life, not to mention the unwelcome weight gain and changes in body temperature. I was frustrated because I couldn't attribute these changes to anything different in my diet or lifestyle. I was desperate to figure out what was going on, and more importantly, what I could do about it.

The stress of building my practice and business, having a family, being president of the California Association of Naturopathic Physicians, and having an overall unrelentingly stressful lifestyle was taking a toll. I had moved back to one of the most polluted—yet beautiful—areas in California. And my dietary choices tended to be less than ideal in times of stress when I needed quick energy. I was drinking coffee in the morning to get me going and looking forward to a glass or two of wine on the weekends so I could finally relax. I was completely out of balance.

My stress level was taxing my adrenal glands. I developed digestive disturbances, which I knew were compromising my liver's ability to do its many jobs, including processing and neutralizing hormones. The effects on my body were manifesting in the form of annoying and uncomfortable symptoms. I knew the last thing I needed was more estrogen from birth control pills. I needed to get my body back in balance. If I didn't work to correct some things, I knew I was increasing my risk down the road for dangerous health conditions, such as cancer.

Listening to the signals my body was sending, such as the difficult periods (which are not normal), then making some profound changes in my diet, lifestyle, and supplement regime got me back on track, in balance, and wiser than before.

What I discovered in treating my patients and myself is that women are experiencing this common collection of symptoms because all of their hormones—not just estrogen and progesterone—are out of balance. This imbalance throws off other bodily systems. Most important, treatment with synthetic hormones is not helping women live longer, healthier lives. Most of these conditions, including difficult transitions to menopause, can be traced to hormone imbalance; more hormones are the last thing women need. In fact, this course of action could be harmful. Hormone imbalance can not only cause the symptoms mentioned above, but also can lead to cancer, heart disease, osteoporosis, and Alzheimer's disease.

Women's hormone health did not become more problematic overnight. It has a lot to do with our modern environment and lifestyles. Pollution, stress, food quality, and prevailing medical practices take their toll on bodily systems. The good news is once we understand what creates imbalance, we can tap the many safe ways of restoring balance and eliminating uncomfortable, irritating symptoms while preventing disease and increasing overall quality of life and well-being.

CHAPTER I

Hormones 101

"Touch one strand and the whole web trembles." —*Deepak Chopra, MD*

O ur bodies are brilliant and built to stay in balance through the harmonious efforts of many interrelated systems. These systems, including the nervous and endocrine systems, work with internal and external influences to keep our bodies functioning on an even keel. The nervous system works with electrical impulses and neurons to adapt to stimuli, and the endocrine system uses chemical messengers called hormones to affect bodily activities. Hormones are powerful messengers that travel through the blood to stimulate a response or cause a reaction. These two systems are intimately related and their activities coordinated. For example, the nervous system can stimulate or inhibit hormone release via the endocrine system.

You can think of hormones as keys and receptors as locks. When a key is placed in a compatible lock, the cell receives instructions to perform a task related to that specific hormone. We used to think only one key worked for each lock, but now we know many keys can fit into the same lock. This is beneficial information, because of all those interchangeable keys, some are helpful and some are harmful. Phytoestrogens, or plant-based hormones, are helpful keys. These can fill receptor sites and block cells from being stimulated by stronger hormones. Harmful hormonal keys, most often from man-made sources such as pesticides and pollution, can stimulate toxic cellular behavior.

Although the best-known hormones—estrogen and progesterone—play a significant role in women's health, the endocrine system produces a variety of other hormones, including cortisol, thymosin, melatonin, glucagon, calcitonin, and thyroxine. Hormones initiate bodily activities when they attach to receptors on the surfaces of cells. They deliver messages. For example, when the uterus is stimulated by estrogen, cells grow and proliferate to create a nourishing lining in preparation for pregnancy.

SPECIALIZED GLANDS

The endocrine system glands are located throughout the body and are intricately related. Each gland secretes hormones that help maintain balance by altering the physiological activities of an organ's cells or of cells in organ groups. Hormones also may directly affect the activities of all the body's cells, such as the thyroid hormone's effects on metabolism. The body's need for any particular hormone determines how much is released. The glands and hormones influence each other and all aspects of growth and development. The system is built with some redundancies for safety and efficiency. All this interconnection is what makes the endocrine system both powerful and vulnerable. Because endocrine activity influences the entire body, healthy endocrine gland function is paramount.

Hypothalamus. Located in the brain, the hypothalamus can be considered the CEO of the endocrine system. It provides direction to the other glands and controls their activity. The hypothalamus is involved in controlling water balance, sugar and fat metabolism, body temperature, and the secretion of releasing and inhibiting hormones.

Pituitary. The pituitary gland is also located in the brain. The hormones it secretes—including follicle-stimulating hormone (FSH) and luteinizing hormone (LH)—help regulate reproduction, growth, and thyroid function. Most tissues in the body are influenced by the pituitary gland.

Pineal. The primary function of this small gland located in the brain is to release melatonin, which helps regulate the daily rhythms of sleep and wakefulness.

Thymus. Sometimes referred to as the master gland of immunity, the thymus is located in the neck. It is intricately involved with immune system development and function.

Pancreas. This gland is located behind the stomach. It works closely with the liver, and its primary function is to help control blood sugar levels. It secretes pancreatic fluid and contributes to digestion of all foods in the small intestine.

Adrenal. Located on the upper portion of the kidneys, these glands are controlled by the sympathetic nervous system and func-

THE ENDOCRINE GLANDS

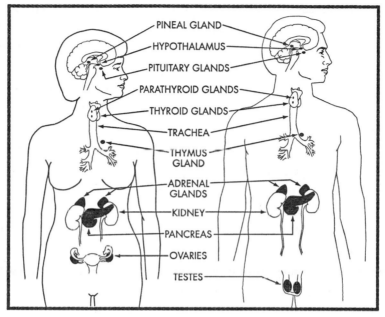

tion in conjunction with it. They adjust bodily responses to stress and emotional changes by releasing norepinephrine and epinephrine. Another part of the adrenal gland secretes other hormones, including cortisol, estrogens, and progestins.

Thyroid. The thyroid is a bow-shaped gland located just below the voice box. It controls metabolism and many other bodily functions. The thyroid gland secretes calcitonin, which is important for maintaining a dense, strong bone matrix and regulating blood calcium levels.

Parathyroid. These small endocrine glands located near the thyroid secrete parathyroid hormones, which regulate calcium and phosphorus metabolism.

Ovaries. These two glands produce eggs and two known hormones, estrogen and progesterone. The ovaries are almond shaped and are located on either side of the pelvic cavity, attached to the uterus by ligaments. FSH and LH primarily control ovarian activity.

Testes. These glands are located in the scrotum and produce sperm and the male hormones testosterone and inhibin.

The hormone messengers are controlled by the endocrine system, which comprises the adrenal, hypothalamus, pancreas, pineal, pituitary, reproductive (testes and ovaries), thyroid, and thymus glands. Their harmonious activities have a significant effect on overall health. If any one of these glands isn't able to function properly because of stress, lifestyle, or dietary influences, the effects are far-reaching and felt body-wide. For example, hormones secreted by the pituitary, thyroid, and ovaries stimulate bone growth. Without the proper amounts of these hormones, bones can become weak, which increases osteoporosis risk. An unhealthy or unbalanced endocrine system can also tax the digestive system, creating ulcers, constipation, or diarrhea. If the endocrine system can't send the proper messages to the thymus gland, the immune system may become compromised, increasing susceptibility to illnesses.

When the endocrine system is functioning properly, there is internal harmony. The endocrine system is designed to maintain balance by using a variety of complex feedback loops. Through numerous internal reactions, the endocrine glands diligently attempt to maintain or create balance through a woman's hormonal stages—puberty, ovulation, menstruation, pregnancy, perimenopause, and menopause.

LIFE CYCLES

Puberty defines the onset of our hormonal cycles and generally occurs between the ages of 9 and 16. In addition to stimulating growth in breast tissue, body hair, and overall height, female puberty is characterized by the onset of menstruation—the monthly discharge of the uterine fluid in the absence of pregnancy.

A typical menstrual cycle lasts about 28 days but can vary from woman to woman. The menstrual cycle's purpose is to stimulate the ovaries to release an egg for possible fertilization and the uterine lining to prepare for possible implantation of that fertilized egg. Estrogen and progesterone are the two predominant hormones driving this process. The menstrual cycle is an excellent example of how connected and intricate the endocrine system is.

The steps of a typical menstrual cycle:
1. The hypothalamus signals the pituitary to release FSH, which causes the ovaries to secrete estrogen so the egg can mature.
2. When estrogen reaches a specific level, the hypothalamus tells the

MENSTRUAL CYCLE

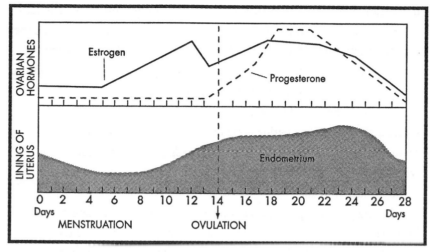

pituitary to secrete LH, which stimulates the release of a fully developed egg. The release of an egg is called ovulation.

3. Estrogen levels then fall as progesterone levels rise to help build the uterine lining to prepare it for the fertilized egg.

4. If the egg is not fertilized after 13 to 15 days, estrogen and progesterone levels both drop, and menstruation begins.

5. The process starts anew.

A balance of estrogen and progesterone levels is necessary for healthy ovulation and menstruation to occur each month. In a normal cycle, estrogen dominates the first half of the cycle until ovulation; progesterone dominates the second half until menstruation.

The dynamic interplay between estrogen and progesterone is extremely important to women's overall health and hormonal balance. Remember, estrogen's primary function is to cause cells to multiply and grow. In the case of normal menstruation, cell growth is a safe and necessary component. However, excessive cell or tissue growth stimulated by excess estrogen is unhealthy and can lead to conditions such as PMS, endometriosis, fibroids, or even cancer. To keep estrogen levels in check, the endocrine system allows progesterone levels to rise and fall, creating a balance. If stress or other factors tax the endocrine system, hormones can get out of balance, leading to all manner of symptoms and disorders.

Another natural part of a woman's hormonal life cycle is menopause, or the cessation of menstruation. As a woman approaches this phase, she may begin feeling hormonal fluctuations when she is as young as 35, though they typically begin three to six years before her last period. This transition between reproductive years and menopause is commonly called premenopause or perimenopause. It is characterized by hormone fluctuations more resembling puberty's wild ride than the rhythmic hormonal flow of the reproductive years. The perimenopausal experience can be subtle or dramatic, depending on heredity, health, stress levels, diet, lifestyle, and whether or not hormones were manipulated with birth control pills during the reproductive years.

During perimenopause, symptoms such as menstrual irregularities, breast tenderness, clouded thinking, weight gain, insomnia, and moodiness may appear as a result of altered hormone activity. As the reproductive years wind down, the ovaries don't always produce an egg every month. (A cycle without ovulation is called an anovulatory cycle.) Without ovulation, the ovaries don't produce progesterone, which leaves estrogen unopposed or unbalanced, and this is attributed to many perimenopausal symptoms.

Menopause begins for the majority of women in their mid-40s to early 50s; the average age is 51. Paramount among the hormonal changes is that the ovaries stop producing estrogen and progesterone. When this happens, menstruation ceases and women may experience other changes as well, including hot flashes, vaginal dryness, mood swings, insomnia, and night sweats, to name a few.

The production of estrogen and progesterone does not stop completely at menopause, but the primary sources of these hormones shift. When the ovaries cease production of these hormones, the adrenal glands and fat cells take over. The body is designed to accommodate this natural process, just as it is able to adjust to puberty and pregnancy.

WHEN SOMETHING'S WRONG

From puberty through fertility to menopause, the flow of a woman's hormones, especially estrogen and progesterone, affect every cell in her body. Estrogen and progesterone are considered sex hormones, because they are so intimately involved in our reproductive cycle. However, in addition to reproduction, these hormones influence bone, heart, brain, and skin health.

That's why when the endocrine or other bodily systems are out of balance, we can have so many different symptoms, ranging from stiff joints, brain fog, and weight gain to PMS and hot flashes.

Symptoms are our bodies' way of sending us messages. They signal something is going on internally. Symptoms of hormonal imbalance, such as mood swings, bloating, hot flashes, and insomnia, are direct messages from the endocrine system that something is changing, that balance has been disrupted. It's important to pay attention to those messages and not just cover them up or drown them out.

Think of symptoms as a smoke alarm in your home. Once activated, the alarm won't subside until the source of the smoke is extinguished. Just treating the symptoms of an illness is like disconnecting a fire alarm instead of extinguishing the fire. Sure, it stops the alarm's irritating noise, but somewhere a fire is still smoldering. If we have symptoms, we must address the source.

Unfortunately, many women have been led to believe their varied hormone-related symptoms, especially during menopause, are caused by estrogen deficiency and should be treated with HRT. However, most health symptoms and conditions can be linked directly or indirectly to an internal environment of estrogen dominance. It is a case of too much estrogen and not enough progesterone—the exact opposite of what women are being told. Prescribing additional estrogen fuels the flame. We must endeavor to keep our endocrine systems functioning effectively so hormonal disruption and the symptoms and illnesses it can cause are mitigated. To successfully ease symptoms and avoid conditions such as osteoporosis and heart disease, we must address the underlying cause of estrogen dominance and overall imbalance.

Addressing the Underlying Cause

Hormones are the potent chemical messengers that keep the body functioning properly. However, the same substances the endocrine glands rely on for efficient communication also can contribute to dysfunction if the system is out of balance in any way. Even small amounts of errant hormonal activity—whether from a stressed organ (the liver, for example), gland (maybe the adrenals), or system (digestive perhaps), or from an external source—can create a profound negative effect.

UNDERSTANDING ESTROGEN

Among the most powerful classes of hormones the body produces is estrogen. Although we commonly think of estrogen as one substance or one type of hormone, it is actually a class of naturally occurring sex hormones produced by the ovaries and the adrenal glands. There are at least two dozen known estrogens, all with various functions; every organ, including the brain, heart, ovaries, and liver, has estrogen-sensitive receptor sites. The most commonly discussed estrogens are estrone, estradiol, and estriol.

Estrone is converted from estradiol primarily in the liver and in fat cells from the precursor hormones androstenedione, progesterone, and dehydroepiandrosterone (DHEA). Estradiol, the principal estrogen, is produced in the ovaries from cholesterol. It has the ability to convert to estrone and back to estradiol in the small intestine. Estradiol is considerably more potent and has been known for decades to be more carcinogenic than the others. It is metabolized into either 2 alpha-hydroxyestrone or 16 alpha-hydroxyestrone. If more 2 hydroxyestrone (an anticancerous agent) is produced, then less 16 hydroxyestrone is made. The 16 hydroxyestrone is more potent than estradiol; it increases cellular growth and can cause cancer in estrogen-sensitive tissues. The third estrogen, estriol, is a bit different from the others in that it cannot be converted to anything after it is formed. There is still some speculation about where estriol comes from. Some believe estradiol and estrone convert to estriol in the liver. Others theorize the ovaries and adrenals secrete it.

The main function of estrogens, as a group, is to promote cell proliferation. They stimulate endometrial cells in preparation for pregnancy, prompt breast tissue growth, maintain function of the sexual organs, stimulate the menstrual cycle, and initiate the bodily changes that occur at puberty. If estrogen function is unchecked, cells can multiply unnecessarily, leading to dangerous situations, such as cancer in some cases. One of the body's hormone mediators for estrogen is progesterone.

Progesterone is one specific hormone, not a group; it is made by the corpus luteum, a part of the ovary, beginning before ovulation and increasing after an egg is released. This hormone is dominant in the latter half of the menstrual cycle. The adrenal glands also produce small amounts of progesterone. Progesterone is carried in the blood and used by the body or excreted after passing through the liver. The three main functions of progesterone are promoting the healthy development of an embryo and fetus, providing a variety of bodily effects (normalizing blood sugar and clotting, maintaining cell oxygenation, acting as a natural antidepressant, protecting against breast and endometrial cancer, among others), and acting as a precursor for other steroid hormones, including estrogen and testosterone. A vitally important feature is that progesterone counteracts estrogen's effects. Whereas estrogen triggers an action, progesterone controls or normalizes that action. For example, estrogen allows water and sodium to flood cells, causing water retention and elevated blood pressure. Progesterone, conversely, acts as a mild diuretic. These hormones work in tandem to keep the body's functions in balance.

Estrogens produced in the body are not the only ones we are exposed to, however. There are estrogens in the air we breathe, the water we drink, and the foods we eat. Many women also take synthetic hormones. Among all the estrogens we come in contact with daily, there are beneficial and detrimental ones. Knowing the sources of these estrogens is helpful in creating hormone balance in your body.

DETRIMENTAL ESTROGENS

We live awash in environmental xenoestrogens that negatively affect our health. They are everywhere. Xenoestrogens are foreign substances with estrogenlike effects in the body. It is important to note that their estrogenic activity is much more potent than the estrogen made by ovaries. Xenoestrogens can mimic natural estrogen or block it at estrogen receptor sites on cells throughout the body. These artificial estrogens activate receptors to stimulate a hormonal effect or occupy the receptor and block natural hormones from doing their job, either way disrupting normal endocrine activity. Many of these hormone imposters accumulate over time because they are fat soluble; they are easily absorbed through the skin and can be stored in body fat, where they can continue to interfere with the body's natural hormone balance.

These man-made estrogens find their way into the water supply, soil, air, and the food chain. As you might imagine, these have a serious effect on hormone balance. Most xenoestrogens are derived from petrochemicals and include pesticides, industrial chemicals, cleaners, plastics (water bottles, food containers), nail polish, and car exhaust. The pollution from these products causes health problems, including increased cancer rates and infertility.

REDUCING XENOESTROGENS IN YOUR LIFE

Xenoestrogens are all around us—that's a fact. Previously, their small amounts of estrogenic activity were dismissed, but recent findings published in *Environmental Health Perspectives* indicate all those little exposures add up. The researchers found that the effects of a collection of xenoestrogens, even though each one was beneath the levels at which they cause an effect, was to more than double the effect of natural estrogen by itself. How do you keep these minute exposures from making a difference in your health? Do what you can to minimize your exposure to xenoestrogens—you'll find them in some unlikely places.

• Avoid plastics for water and food storage. Use glass or ceramics whenever possible, especially to heat food. When plastic is heated, it rapidly diffuses into food. Use wax paper or a glass plate instead of plastic wrap to cover bowls in the microwave.

- Use detergents with fewer chemicals. Chemical residue can be absorbed through your skin.
- Choose shampoos, body soaps, makeup, and lotions that are paraben free.
- Use natural pest control, not pesticides or herbicides.
- Buy hormone-free meats; look for organics whenever possible.
- Buy organic produce to reduce your exposure to herbicides, pesticides, and other chemicals.
- Avoid birth control pills, spermicides, and HRT.

In a recent study published in the journal *Occupational and Environmental Medicine,* researchers made a direct link between cancer and pesticides. Women with breast cancer were five times more likely to have pesticide residue in their bloodstream than healthy women were.

Synthetic hormones, in the form of birth control pills and HRT, introduce other man-made estrogens and provide another means of disrupting hormone balance, and as a result, health. These commercial hormones are structurally altered and different from the ones we produce. The list of risks related to taking synthetic hormones is long. Women taking birth control pills are at increased risk for high blood pressure and blood clots. Clotting can lead to sometimes-fatal strokes, heart attacks, or pulmonary emboli, depending on where the clot develops. Other serious adverse reactions, as listed in the *Physicians' Desk Reference* (Medical Economics Co., 2003), include gallbladder disease and breast, liver, and endometrial cancer. Patients using oral contraceptives have reported numerous adverse reactions, including breast changes, colitis, congenital abnormalities, depression, impaired kidney function, menstrual changes, and weight changes.

Not all estrogens are bad, though. Our bodies require this hormone for proper functioning, but it should be the estrogen naturally created in our bodies, and it should be present in proper proportion with progesterone and other natural hormones. Balance is the key. There are also "good" external estrogens, namely those from plants, which we acquire from our diet. These beneficial estrogens can act as allies in reinstating or maintaining hormone balance.

BENEFICIAL ESTROGENS

Phytoestrogens are plant-based substances with weak estrogenic activity. They are considered hormone balancers because they have both mild estrogenic and antiestrogenic effects. They can compete with the more potent estrogens discussed above by vying for receptor sites on cells. By occupying these sites, phytoestrogens can limit the activity of more potent natural estrogens, as well as xenoestrogens. They provide a balancing effect based on what the body needs. If there is too much estrogen, phytoestrogens will block estrogenic activity. If the body does not have enough estrogen, phytoestrogens will provide mild estrogenic activity.

Phytoestrogens can be found in foods including flaxseeds, legumes (soybeans, lentils, and chickpeas, for example), fennel, celery, and parsley. They are also present in various herbs, including alfalfa (*Medicago sativa*), chaste tree berry (*Vitex angus-castus*), dong quai (*Angelica sinensis*), sage (*Salvia officinalis*), hops (*Humulus lupulus*), red clover (*Trifolium pratense*), and wild yam (*Dioscorea villosa*).

In a study published in the *Journal of the National Cancer Institute* in 2003, researchers evaluated the associations between dietary intake of phytoestrogens and endometrial cancer risk. What they found was that consumption of isoflavone and lignan (a phytoestrogen present in legumes and flaxseeds) was inversely related to endometrial cancer risk. Obese postmenopausal women consuming relatively low amounts of phytoestrogens had the highest endometrial cancer risk.

ESTROGEN METABOLISM

Phytoestrogens are metabolized in the intestinal tract where they are converted into their active form, meaning they are biologically available to tissues and then absorbed. Optimal digestion—specifically bacterial balance in the intestinal tract—is critical, because an overgrowth of harmful bacteria will inhibit the effectiveness of phytoestrogens by disrupting the necessary conversion process.

Estrogen, on the other hand, is metabolized in the liver. Proper estrogen metabolism keeps the body's estrogen content in balance. The liver rids the body of excess hormones by secreting chemicals to disarm them so they can be eliminated. One way the liver removes excess hormones is to produce glucuronic acid. This compound attaches to the hormone, creating a new, harmless substance that can be eliminated from the body.

Unfortunately, this process is easily disrupted by a poor diet. Eating too much sugar and red meat can cause the release of a bacterial enzyme in the gut, known as beta-glucuronidase. This enzyme cleaves the bond between the glucuronic acid and estrogen, which means the intact hormone molecule can continue to circulate. Without the beta-glucuronidase attachment, estrogen can't be eliminated, so it is reabsorbed into the bloodstream. It may return to the liver several times before being eliminated. This inefficiency strains the liver, not allowing it to effectively perform its many other tasks.

One way to ascertain the efficiency of your estrogen metabolism is with a blood or urine test. Great Smokies Diagnostic Laboratories (www.gsdl.com) offers blood and urine estrogen metabolism assessment tests that evaluate how estrogen is being processed in the body. Results will reveal hormonal imbalances that can increase risk of estrogen-dependent health conditions, including breast cancer, lupus, osteoporosis, and heart disease. Results will also show the physiological effects of hormone therapy, so interventions can be adjusted if necessary. Armed with this information, you and your health-care provider can make better decisions about restoring hormone balance in your body. With more-than-necessary amounts of estrogen in the body, a condition commonly called estrogen dominance develops.

ESTROGEN DOMINANCE

When there is an excess of any hormone, an imbalance develops, and health problems can arise. When there is too much estrogen and not enough progesterone to counteract its effects, the situation is called estrogen dominance. Estrogen dominance is caused by exposure to excess environmental xenoestrogens, use of synthetic estrogens (birth control pill and HRT), anovulation (lack of ovulation during menstrual cycle, which is not uncommon among women older than 35), digestion issues (which tax the estrogen-detoxification process in the liver), unrelenting stress (which strains the adrenals and the thyroid), poor diet, unresolved emotional issues, and negative lifestyle factors (including smoking).

How does estrogen dominance specifically alter women's health? It has been linked to a wide range of conditions, including PMS, uterine fibroids, and endometriosis, as well as symptoms including allergies, decreased libido, fatigue, fibrocystic breasts, headaches, infertility, irritability, and fat gain. In addition, numerous studies demonstrate excess estrogen can cause breast, uterine, and ovarian cancers (which are all considered estrogen-dependent cancers), and cervical dysplasia (a precancerous condition characterized by abnormal changes to cervical tissues).

In a study published in 2000 in the journal *Gynecologic Oncology*, researchers identified hormone replacement, particularly unopposed estrogens after hysterectomy, as a significant risk factor for endometrial cancer. Researchers also noticed a trend for increased risk among obese women. They say hyperestrogenism (excess estrogen), either from external sources or created in the body, is a significant risk factor for cancer from endometriosis.

THE DANGERS OF ESTROGEN DOMINANCE

It is easy to see how, in our contemporary lifestyles, estrogen can begin to dominate the hormone scene, with the prevalence of xenoestrogens; the use of HRT and oral contraceptives; diets skewed in favor of nonorganic fruits, vegetables, meats, and dairy products (which frequently contain xenoestrogens); stressful lifestyles; and increased estrogen production because of anovulation, imbalanced ovarian function, and hysterectomies. Estrogen dominance can manifest in numerous ways, including PMS, headaches, fatigue, fat gain around the abdomen, decreased libido, acceleration of the aging process, cervical dysplasia, uterine fibroids, and uterine and breast cancer.

Cancer is among the most disconcerting of the possible outcomes of estrogen dominance. Because cancer rates are increasing every decade, it is likely that cancer has touched your life in some profound way. I know I am seeing more women with estrogen-dependent cancers in my clinical practice than ever before.

The American Cancer Society (ACS) estimates one in three women will develop some type of cancer in her lifetime. Breast cancer rates have increased from one in 20 in 1960 to one in eight today, though the rates have slowed since the 1990s. But the ACS says breast cancer incidence rates have increased lately in women older than 50. Among the risks the ACS lists for breast cancer are long menstrual history (early onset of menses and late menopause) and use of oral contraceptives and postmenopausal estrogens and progestin. These risk factors increase the lifetime exposure to estrogen.

The connection between excess estrogen and certain cancers is clear. Harmful estrogens are difficult to detoxify and are stored in fat. In a recent study published in the *Journal of the National Cancer Institute*, researchers linked obesity to breast cancer. Women with a higher body mass index (BMI), which equated to higher levels of body fat, also had elevated hormone levels, particularly of estradiol, which is the more potent of the estrogens produced in the body. The researchers concluded, "The increase in breast cancer risk with increasing BMI among postmenopausal women is largely the result of the associated increase in estrogens, particularly bioavailable estradiol."

According to a study featured in *Cancer Causes and Control,* women can reduce their breast cancer risk by maintaining a normal weight, because that reduces the amount of hormones stored in fat.

Given this knowledge, it is troublesome that HRT is so frequently prescribed for perimenopause and menopause. Fortunately, recent broad media attention regarding the Women's Health Initiative (WHI) study has helped educate the general public. The WHI was designed to prove the effectiveness of a popular HRT drug known as Prempro (a combination of synthetic estrogen from the urine of pregnant mares and progestin). The study was stopped early, because the drug posed such a danger to the participants. Results indicated women taking the drug were at a significantly higher risk of developing invasive breast cancer and ovarian cancer than women not taking the drug. In addition to cancer, the WHI demonstrated that prescription HRT significantly increased the risk of blood clots and heart disease.

According to results of the Nurses' Health Study, the risk of developing cancer increases dramatically with HRT use. Consider the following statistics from the Harvard Medical School's 16-year study in which researchers followed 122,000 nurses.

36—How many times more likely women taking estrogen are to develop breast cancer than those who aren't.

50 percent—The increased likelihood of developing breast cancer among women taking estrogen and progestin.

60 percent—How much higher the risk of ovarian cancer is among women who took HRT compared with women who did not.

71 percent—The increase in breast cancer rates among women between the ages of 60 and 64 who took HRT for five years or more.

78 percent—The increase in risk for developing breast cancer among those taking estrogen and testosterone.

240 percent—The increase in breast cancer rates among women taking progestins alone.

SUPPLEMENTAL HELP FOR HORMONE BALANCE

Several natural remedies for helping to clear excess estrogen can help you bring your hormones back into balance. Discuss the following with your healthcare provider.

D-glucarate is a botanical substance found in many fruits and vegetables, including grapefruit, apples, oranges, broccoli, and brussels sprouts. **Calcium D-glucarate**, the calcium salt form, is marketed as a nutritional supplement. This compound appears to protect against cancer and other diseases. Calcium D-glucarate slows the release of a substance that inhibits glucuronidase, which is an enzyme that interferes with the body's efforts to eliminate cancer-causing substances known as carcinogens. Results of studies show this compound to have preventive and therapeutic activity against a number of cancers, including breast, liver, prostate, and colon. Researchers have demonstrated that calcium D-glucarate contributes to healthy cell development and estrogen metabolism. In animal studies, calcium D-glucarate reduced blood levels of estradiol, the form of estrogen that causes breast cancer. Researchers conclude D-glucarate lowers the level of glucuronidase, thus allowing the body to eliminate harmful carcinogens. The typical dose is 200 mg once or twice daily.

You can find another natural estrogen detoxifier in cruciferous vegetables, such as broccoli, cauliflower, brussels sprouts, and cabbage. Known as **indole-3-carbinol (I3C)**, this compound has been shown in clinical studies to help the body detoxify excess estrogens. Many studies conclude that I3C can help prevent estrogen-dependent cancers such as breast, ovarian, and uterine.

In one study conducted at New York Medical College, researchers showed I3C inhibited the activity of the potent estrogen, 17 beta-estradiol (E2). Excess E2 is a known cause of breast cancer. In another study involving women with lupus, an autoimmune condition also associated with poor estrogen metabolism, researchers demonstrated I3C could help reduce disease symptoms.

The drawback of I3C is that it is considered an unstable molecule. To be effective, it must be converted into **diindolymethane (DIM)** in the body. As far as supplements go, I recommend DIM versus I3C for these reasons:

- Because I3C is unstable, its absorption is unpredictable and it is not biologically active if it is not converted to DIM.

- You would need to take 30 times more I3C than DIM because of its unpredictable absorption rate.
- High doses of I3C can cause dizziness and gastritis, whereas no such effects have been found with DIM. High IC3 doses also are associated with altered detoxification metabolism.

Although I3C shows some promise in the scientific literature, DIM appears to be the safer and more effective choice. Both I3C and DIM are available as dietary supplements. DIM has been shown to provide relief from PMS, painful periods, and breast tenderness. Higher doses improve cervical dysplasia and weight loss. IC3 hasn't been shown to do any of these. DIM helps reduce levels of the dangerous 16 hydroxyestrone and increase levels of the protective 2 hydroxyestrone. A daily dose of 30 mg of bioactive, supplemental DIM is equivalent to eating two pounds of broccoli. DIM helps support a healthy balance of hormones by promoting the breakdown and excretion of excess estrogens associated with certain types of cancer.

Estrogen dominance is also associated with low progesterone levels, so it is important to consider ways to enhance levels of this hormone. One of the most widely used herbal extracts to positively influence progesterone production is **chaste tree** (*Vitex agnus-castus*). According to the *PDR for Herbal Medicines* (Thomson Healthcare, 2000), chaste tree has historically been used to relieve menstrual problems. In Europe, chaste tree extract is an approved treatment for PMS and menstrual irregularities. Chaste tree stimulates the pituitary gland to produce more LH, which stimulates progesterone production. The recommended daily dose is 20 to 25 mg.

Over-the-counter and prescription **progesterone creams** are also available. Although these creams can provide benefit, they must be used as directed and are typically more effective when monitored by a healthcare professional. I have seen patients who experience positive results and then either consciously or subconsciously start using more of the cream, thinking more is better. This can contribute to imbalance rather than repair it. I typically don't recommend progesterone cream to my patients, because my philosophy is to lean toward restoring function rather than replacing it.

Another option is a **castor oil pack**. This traditional treatment is often prescribed for hormone imbalance, intestinal disorders, liver and gallbladder conditions, headaches, urinary tract infections, and cleansing/detoxification programs. To make a castor oil pack, saturate a piece of wool or cotton flannel with cold-pressed castor oil. Alternately place the oil-saturated cloth directly on the abdomen and over the liver. Cover the pack with plastic and apply heat, typically in the form of a hot water bottle. Don't use castor oil packs during pregnancy or the heaviest days of your menstrual cycle. Relax with this treatment in place for one hour up to three times a week. Castor oil packs can also be used once weekly as preventive medicine. The oil is absorbed into circulation, providing a cleansing, nutritive, and relaxing treatment. This treatment has been shown to increase immune system function and improve hormone balance by stimulating the liver to clear excess hormones.

ALTERING THE COURSE

The issue of estrogen dominance is a key cause of many symptoms and conditions women face today. To relieve symptoms and avoid illness, it is important to address the underlying causes rather than simply mask symptoms. Often the underlying cause is estrogen imbalance. We can reduce the cancer risk of an estrogen-dominant internal environment by correcting the underlying imbalance. In addition to maintaining a healthy diet and lifestyle, reduce exposure to xenoestrogens, avoid prescription estrogens, enhance estrogen metabolism, and emphasize beneficial estrogens (phytoestrogens).

CHAPTER 3

Importance of a Strong Foundation

The foundation of health is built on wise dietary choices, prudent supplementation, regular exercise, and an awareness of mind/body/emotion connection. With attention to these four elements, you give your body the best possible chance to stay healthy and in balance, increasing your odds of living a long, healthy life.

THE FOOD FACTOR

Every biochemical action on a cellular level is fueled by a vitamin or mineral cofactor. Vitamins, minerals, enzymes, and amino acids fuel our bodies to keep us healthy and active. Even marginal nutritional deficiencies can limit our vitality, compromise our immunity, and damage our health. This means our food selections are of utmost importance. Other than vitamin D, which is converted from sunshine by our skin, we get all the vital nutrients we need from food or dietary supplements; we don't make them.

Every day we make dietary choices that either positively or negatively affect our health. It is important to understand the connection between what we eat and how we feel. The best way to improve health is to make dietary and lifestyle changes that last a lifetime and not flit from plan to plan with each diet book of the moment. The philosophy I share with my patients isn't unique. It is a commonsense approach emphasizing foods that nourish and habits that encourage positive lifestyle choices. Understanding the deficiencies of the standard American diet should help you see the importance of reconstructing your shopping and eating habits.

STANDARD AMERICAN DIET

The typical American diet emphasizes quantity rather than quality. It is notoriously high in calories and woefully low in nutritional value. Jacob

Teitelbaum, MD, author of *From Fatigued to Fantastic* (Avery Penguin Putnam, 2001), calls the problem high-calorie malnutrition. "It is not just our affection for fast food, super-sized portions, and mega 'big-burp' sodas," he says, "It is also the fact that the processed foods we rely on have been sucked dry of so many nutrients." According to the 1998 Teen Eating Study, teenagers eat at fast food restaurants at least twice a week—a habit costing them $13 billion a year. The U.S. Department of Agriculture reported that, every year, the average American consumes more than 120 pounds of sugar, 115 pounds of red meat, 53 gallons of carbonated soft drinks, 16 pounds of ice cream, and nearly 1,100 cups of coffee.

The National Health and Nutrition Survey (NHANES 1999) says in the past two decades the number of overweight Americans has nearly doubled. "The nutrition transition towards refined foods, foods of animal origin, and increased fats plays a major role in current global epidemics of obesity, diabetes, and cardiovascular disease," according to the 2002 World Health Organization report on dietary habits.

In addition to obesity, diabetes, and cardiovascular disease, poor nutrition can amplify symptoms of hormone imbalance. When the body does not use the extra sugar consumed for energy, it is converted to fat, where excess hormones are stored. In addition, eating too much sugar can cause a sluggish metabolism and strain the pancreas and liver—organs you need functioning at their peak for proper digestion and hormone metabolism. Symptoms associated with a high-sugar diet can include insomnia, hyperactivity, weight gain, and rebound fatigue after the initial spike in energy. Fatigue is common because the energy from sugar is not sustained, and fatigue leads to more sugar consumption. "Tired people have, as we know, decreased adrenal function and suppressed immune systems, both of which lead the body to crave sugar," Teitelbaum says.

Sugar isn't our only vice. Highly processed foods also contribute to hormone imbalance. The liver processes preservatives, additives, and artificial flavorings. If the liver is too busy metabolizing these substances, it will be unable to process excess estrogens and other toxins, which can lead to estrogen dominance. Symptoms associated with a diet high in preservatives, additives, and artificial flavorings and colorings can include foggy thinking, headaches, anxiety, and depression.

So if we endeavor to remove many of the empty calories and artificial ingredients from our diets and get our nourishment from whole foods, we can help our bodies function at optimal performance levels. Think of it as good fuel for a clean-running machine.

MAKING HEALTHY CHOICES

Proactive meal planning is such an important part of reworking your dietary habits. By planning, you will have the foods you need at home to pack a lunch or snack and to make healthy breakfasts and dinners. With the right stuff available, you'll be less tempted by those quick and empty options. Here are the core aspects of my commonsense dietary approach.

Eat the colors of the rainbow. Whenever you eat, look at what color your meal is. Is it brown and white or red, green, yellow, and orange? The more colorful your meals, the healthier you will be. Get your color from an assortment of seasonal whole fruits and vegetables. Berries are rich in anti-oxidants; sprinkle some on your morning cereal or blend frozen berries with a banana and soy or rice milk for a delicious smoothie. Experiment with seasonal vegetables by finding new recipes—butternut squash soup in fall, roasted root vegetables in winter, grilled asparagus in spring, a different salad every few days during summer. An Asian stir fry is a quick and easy meal and a great opportunity for color (think red, yellow and green bell peppers; orange carrots; purple cabbage; plus a little tofu or lean meat over brown rice). With a little experimentation and practice, you'll find colorful cooking much more satisfying than the quick meal from a box.

Eat five to nine servings of fruits and vegetables daily. The National Cancer Institute and other respected organizations recommend between five and nine servings of fruits and vegetables per day to help prevent serious illness. A serving is equal to one medium-size fruit, one-half cup raw or cooked vegetable, one cup lettuce or spinach, one cup fruit or vegetable juice, or one-quarter cup dried fruit. Nine servings can seem overwhelming, considering the average American is lucky to get three a day. But a little planning can go a long way. You can get three easily just at breakfast if you put one-half cup of applesauce on your oatmeal, drink a cup of juice, and eat a piece of fruit. Pack fruit or vegetable pieces for snacks, choose salads for lunch, and include a vegetable or two at dinner and you should be covered. The effort pays off in more ways than one. A diet rich in fruits and vegetables provides fiber, antioxidant nutrients, phytochemicals, and essential fatty acids but is low in saturated fat. You'll fill up on quality foods instead of bouncing from one calorie-laden snack to another. You'll feel better, probably lose a few pounds, and you'll be reducing your risk of cancer, heart disease, hormone imbalance, and other chronic degenerative diseases.

Pay attention to shopping habits. Try to shop several times a week and buy more perishable items rather than stocking up once a week or every other week on processed packaged foods. Shop on the store's periphery, avoiding inner aisles where the canned, preservative-filled packages reside. The freshest, most wholesome foods are located on the perimeter of most grocery stores. Don't shop when you're hungry, and always carry a shopping list based on your menu plan.

Eat whole foods. This means foods in their natural form, not foods filled with additives, preservatives, colors, and chemicals. Avoid ingredients with the word artificial before them. Synthetic food additives have been linked to depression, asthma, allergies, migraine headaches, and, in children, hyperactivity and learning disabilities. Of course, these additives tax the liver, which is charged with processing and clearing these unnatural ingredients from the body. To help you rethink some foods that may find their way into your grocery cart too often, consider how far a food has gone from its most natural form. Eat foods as close to their original state as possible. If it can't run, swim, or be picked at a farm, think twice about eating it.

Drink water. Water is vital for proper internal cellular and organ function. Our bodies are more than 60 percent water by weight. To keep your body lubricated and functioning properly, drink half your body weight in ounces each day (this means a 120-pound person should aim for 60 ounces of water a day). If this seems overwhelming, try carrying a water bottle. Putting it in your way will remind you of your intention. Not drinking enough water stresses the body and can affect kidney function. If you don't like how your tap water tastes, consider a filtration system. Other ways to jazz up your water: add a slice of lemon or lime, put in a splash of juice, or brew a decaffeinated herbal tea and drink up.

Be mindful of how much you eat and when you eat. Most restaurant portions today are enough for two or three meals. Don't think you have to belong to the clean plate club, as mom used to demand. Ask for a to-go box and pack up half your meal right away if you think you'll be tempted to overeat. Portion control is a major factor in cleaning up dietary habits. Even people making good choices often eat too much. In Ayurvedic medicine, an Indian mode of healing, practitioners recommend eating only as much as you can hold in your cupped hands per meal.

The timing of meals is important, too. It is much easier on our bodies if we redistribute our calorie consumption so we are eating more in the morning and less in the evening, when our bodies are trying to wind down. This is often the exact opposite of how many of us eat. When we wake up in the morning, our metabolism is at its highest and most efficient. This is the best time to eat well and provide our bodies with the fuel they need to sustain us throughout the day. Eating too much too late when our metabolism is slow can result in excess body weight, because the unused fuel is stored as fat. Eating smaller meals throughout the day will help normalize blood sugar levels and stabilize metabolism, because a steady supply of fuel is easier to manage than big influxes. Frequent, small meals also encourage healthy digestion, because the body has less food to process at one time.

Balance high-quality protein, fat, and carbohydrates at each meal. Extremes are unhealthy, and an excess of any of these macronutrients can be harmful. A high-protein diet can cause problems with calcium absorption and subsequently impair bone health. If the protein sources aren't lean, the dietary fat can contribute to elevated cholesterol levels, obesity, and gout. Too much fat also can encourage increased estrogen storage. A diet rich in simple carbohydrates can create spikes in blood sugar, resulting in insulin resistance and rebound low blood sugar leading to fatigue and obesity.

Eat organic foods whenever possible. Many studies have now confirmed organic foods contain few, if any, harmful chemicals or xenoestrogens compared with conventionally grown foods. Also, organic foods contain more nutrients. According to a comparison study published in the *Journal of Alternative and Complementary Medicine,* organics are more nutritious. The author concluded, "Organic crops contained significantly more vitamin C, iron, magnesium, and phosphorus and significantly less nitrates than conventional crops. There were nonsignificant trends showing less protein but of a better quality and a higher content of nutritionally significant minerals with lower amounts of some heavy metals in organic crops compared with conventional ones."

According to the Environmental Working Group, a not-for-profit environmental research organization, there is a "dirty dozen" of foods to avoid or only buy in organic form, because they consistently test positive for high pesticide levels. Try to eat organic versions of the following: apples, bell peppers, celery, cherries, imported grapes, nectarines, peaches, pears, potatoes, red raspberries, spinach, and strawberries. The same group found the following 12 to be the least contaminated: asparagus, avocados, bananas, broccoli, cauliflower, corn (sweet), kiwi, mangos, onions, papaya, pineapples, and peas (sweet).

I realize organic foods can sometimes be more expensive, and availability is limited in some areas. If you can't find organic fruits and vegetables, or if they are not within your budget, be sure to wash conventionally grown fruits and vegetables thoroughly before eating them. Just know that some contaminants are designed not to wash off and others are taken up by the fruit or vegetable and can't be washed off. Eat a variety of fruits and vegetables to reduce your exposure to potentially dangerous chemicals found on any particular type.

EATING ORGANICS

According to the National Organic Standards Board, organic farming uses techniques to restore, maintain, and enhance ecological harmony while avoiding pesticides and fertilizers. Organic foods have been processed without artificial ingredients, preservatives, genetically modified ingredients, or irradiation. Fewer chemicals used in farming and food production means fewer chemicals in the environment and in our bodies. Not only are organic foods healthier for the planet, they've proven healthier for those who eat them.

Virginia Worthington, PhD, of Johns Hopkins University says eating organic produce can help prevent nutrient deficiencies. Her study, featured in the *Journal of Alternative and Complementary Medicine*, revealed organically grown foods had 29 percent more magnesium, 27 percent more vitamin C, and 21 percent more iron than conventionally grown foods. Researchers at Truman State University in Missouri found organically grown oranges had up to 30 percent more vitamin C than conventionally grown oranges, even though the organic oranges were smaller.

The popularity of organic foods is increasing. The USDA's Economic Research Service reported in February 2003 that organic products are in nearly 20,000 natural health stores and 73 percent of mainstream grocery stores. Organic product use was up 10 percent from 1999 to 2000. In 2002, nearly 40 percent of the United States population used organic products at least weekly.

Shopping for organics has never been easier. The USDA's national organic standards program has been in effect since October 2002; the program brought clear labeling to products that are 100 percent organic or are made with organic ingredients. Now the term organic means something specific on a food product, making it easier to make informed decisions at the grocery store.

Eat hormone-free beef, milk, chicken, eggs, pork, and fish. It is especially important for women with symptoms of hormonal imbalance or women with a family history of hormone-dependent cancers to eat hormone-free dairy and meat. Most likely, this means eating organic meat, because meat from conventionally raised animals contains higher amounts of xenoestrogens than hormone-free meat products. Conventionally raised animals are exposed to pesticides in their food and often to drug therapy to speed their readiness for slaughter and to maintain their health in often less-than-optimal living conditions. These chemicals make their way into the meat and onto your plate. When it comes to fish, wild-caught fish often contain fewer xenoestrogens than farmed fish. "You are what you eat" applies not only to us, but to everything that eats.

Read labels carefully. It is scientifically documented that trans fats, indicated as hydrogenated oils or partially hydrogenated oils, are harmful. They interfere with the body's ability to use essential fatty acids, and they contribute to cholesterol imbalance. Foods that contain these harmful fats include margarine, chips, crackers, baked goods, and many fast-food restaurant items. Trans fats are produced by heating liquid vegetable oils so they can remain solid at room temperature, which increases product shelf life, but also creates a toxic substance. Hydrogenated or partially hydrogenated oils interfere with the liver's detoxification function and affect immunity. Studies have also shown trans fats increase the risk of type 2 diabetes and heart disease. The *American Journal of Clinical Nutrition* published results of a study in which researchers found an association between trans fat consumption and type 2 diabetes in women. The researchers say substituting nonhydrogenated fatty acids for trans fats would likely reduce the risk of type 2 diabetes substantially. In a study conducted in the Netherlands, researchers examining a population with high trans fat intake concluded this type of diet contributes to coronary heart disease risk. According to their results published in the *Lancet,* decreasing this type of fat intake could have a large public health impact. Finally, in the United States, the FDA has ruled that, by 2006, all trans fats must be listed on food labels, thus allowing shoppers to make informed decisions about what they put in their bodies.

HIDDEN TRANS FATS

Trans fats are often found in processed and convenience foods. Read labels carefully to avoid products containing them. If the ingredient list contains partially hydrogenated vegetable (or corn, soybean, or canola) oil or vegetable shortening, the product contains trans fats. Here are a few common culprits—they may surprise you.

- bread and bread mixes
- breakfast cereals
- cakes and cake mixes
- cookies
- crackers
- donuts
- fried foods in many fast-food restaurants
- frosting
- frozen foods, including hash browns and French fries
- granola bars

- instant soup mixes
- low-fat foods
- margarine
- microwave popcorn
- mixes for sauces, dips, and gravy
- peanut butter
- potato and corn chips
- powdered nondairy coffee creamers
- pudding
- shortening

Not all versions of the above foods contain trans fats, and they certainly don't need to be made with trans fats.

Choose sources of protein and carbohydrates wisely. When choosing sources of protein, consider their fat content. Lean protein contains less saturated fat. Opt for fish, poultry without the skin, and low-fat beef (less than 15 percent fat). But animal products aren't your only options for high-quality protein—don't forget beans, nuts and nut butters, seeds, tofu and other soy-based foods, and some grains and vegetables. Vegetarian protein sources have fiber and no cholesterol, which are dietary bonuses.

Not all carbohydrates are created equal, either. Whole grain breads, cereals, and vegetables are complex carbohydrates. They take longer to digest, so the sugars from these foods enter the bloodstream more slowly than refined sugars do. This keeps blood sugar levels and appetite under control. These carbohydrates are also richer in fiber and vitamins and lower in calories than simple or processed carbohydrates, which include white bread, white flour, candies, cakes, and the like.

The modern lifestyle is no doubt hectic. We are often so busy worrying about our next meeting at work or which bill to pay that we forget to think about our next meal. It is definitely easy to be seduced by convenience rather than health and choose fast over fulfilling. But it is necessary in building a strong foundation to evaluate your daily eating habits, improve where you can, and supplement to fill in any gaps.

THE BENEFITS OF SOY

Soybeans contain quality protein, carbohydrates, oils, and phytoestrogens. Soybeans are particularly rich in a group of phytoestrogens called isoflavones, which have numerous healthy properties. Isoflavones are antioxidants and weak natural estrogens. These isoflavones have been shown to reduce hot flashes in menopausal women, lower cholesterol levels, and reduce the risk of heart disease, osteoporosis, and cancer.

A group of Italian researchers tested soy's ability to reduce hot flashes in postmenopausal women aged 45 to 62. The women added 60 grams of soy protein or casein (to serve as a placebo) to their daily diets for three months. Before the study, all the women experienced at least seven severe hot flashes or night sweats daily. After the study, those eating soy protein reduced their hot flashes by 45 percent.

With regard to heart disease and cholesterol, *The New England*

Journal of Medicine published results of a meta-analysis in which a researcher found dietary soy reduced cholesterol levels in 89 percent of the studies analyzed. The author concluded adding soy to the diet could add up to a 20 percent to 30 percent reduction in heart disease risk. This result bests prescription cholesterol-lowering drugs, if you factor in cost and side effects. The science is so solid for soy and heart disease that the U.S. FDA approved a health claim for soy-based foods stating that adding 25 grams of soy protein per day to a diet low in fat may lower cholesterol and thus heart disease risk. To qualify for the claim, a serving of soy food must contain 6.25 grams of soy protein, less than 3 grams of fat, no more than 1 gram of saturated fat, and less than 20 mg of cholesterol and also be low in sodium.

Soy isoflavones appear to prevent osteoporosis by preventing bone loss. In a study conducted at the University of Cincinnati College of Medicine, researchers found when postmenopausal women added to their daily diet 60 to 70 mg of soy isoflavones, they reduced their bone turnover rate significantly after 12 weeks.

The components of soy can also prevent cancer; they do this in a number of ways, including hormonal effects, cell differentiation, free radical scavenging, and immune stimulation. As I've already discussed, xenoestrogens and high levels of natural estrogens can contribute to cancer. The way soy helps protect against cancer is by filling estrogen receptor sites, which prevents more dangerous estrogens from doing so and thereby reducing cancer risk. In a study, researchers assessed the correlation between phytoestrogen intake and breast cancer risk. The researchers evaluated the diets of subjects with newly diagnosed breast cancer and the same number of cancer-free women. What they found was a substantial reduction in breast cancer risk among women with diets rich in phytoestrogens and the lignans found in soy fiber.

There are numerous ways to increase your soy intake these days. Soy products proliferate in mainstream as well as natural products stores. Look for fresh soy beans (edamame), tofu, marinated and baked tofu, tempeh, miso, textured vegetable protein, soy versions of familiar foods (hot dogs, meatballs, burgers), and soy beverages.

SUPPLEMENTING THE DIET

I take a conservative view of dietary supplementation. I think there is danger in making broad recommendations, because we are all unique; we have individual needs. The scientific literature is very clear, however, that everyone should be taking a high-quality multivitamin/mineral supplement. Recently, results of a landmark meta-analysis featured in *JAMA* (the Journal of the American Medical Association) confirmed that everyone should supplement their diets with vitamins and minerals. The researchers said suboptimal intake of some vitamins is a risk factor for chronic diseases and is common in the general population, especially the elderly. "Suboptimal folic acid levels, along with suboptimal levels of vitamins B6 and B12, are a risk factor for cardiovascular disease, neural tube defects, and colon and breast cancer; low levels of vitamin D contribute to osteopenia and fractures; and low levels of the antioxidant vitamins (vitamins A, E, and C) may increase risk for several chronic diseases," they wrote.

According to the *JAMA* report, there are also subcategories of the population with increased nutrient needs that cannot be met through diet alone. These include menstruating, pregnant, or nursing women; women with a family history of cancer, heart disease, or osteoporosis; people who smoke and/or drink alcohol; the elderly; and vegans. In other words, most people need a multivitamin.

There are other reasons that multivitamins are more of a necessity now. One is that our soil is severely depleted of important nutrients because of overcultivation and increased use of fertilizers and pesticides. The *Journal of Alternative and Complementary Medicine* reported that conventionally grown foods have 32 percent less iron, 29 percent less calcium, and 21 percent less magnesium due, in part, to nutrient-depleted soil. In addition, the *Journal of Agricultural and Food Chemistry* recently reported that conventional farming techniques produce foods that have lower antioxidant activity and therefore cannot as effectively protect us from illness. Another reason multivitamins are a must is that food processing and preservatives, fillers, and other chemicals added to foods remove important nutrients or interfere with their absorption. Artificial colors, for example, interfere with B vitamin absorption and utilization.

When you go looking for a multivitamin, it is important to choose a high-quality dietary supplement. Often, the old adage, "you get what you pay for" applies here, so price should not dictate your decision. If you are going to take a multivitamin, take a good one. Here are some guidelines for choosing dietary supplements:

• Buy supplements made by an established manufacturer with a solid reputation. Find out if the company follows Good Manufacturing Practices (GMPs), which are rules that standardize manufacturing and set clear guidelines for safety, record keeping, sanitation, and ingredient handling. Visit the manufacturer's web site, ask questions about their history, and do a little research about the company before buying their products.

• Be cautious of manufacturers that make aggressive or outlandish claims about their products. If it seems too good to be true, it probably is. These manufacturers are not legally allowed to make unsubstantiated claims for their products, but when they do, the dietary supplements industry loses credibility. Many companies have solid research behind their products, not just slick marketing campaigns.

• Read the label carefully. Avoid products with artificial ingredients such as propylene glycol, sucralose, and talc. Natural, not synthetic, is very important when you are supplementing. Buying products that contain synthetic ingredients defeats the purpose.

• Look for quality rather than quantity. Buy formulations that contain many of the nutrients and herbs you are looking for in one product so you don't have to buy them individually.

• When buying herbal extract products, look for standardized amounts of the active ingredients listed on the label. The entire herb is used, but the product is standardized for a key component so every capsule contains a consistent amount of active ingredient. This provides more predictable results. Many herbs can now be standardized to a particular active compound; often the standardized herb is the one used in the scientific studies.

• Be inquisitive. Ask questions and become a supplement super sleuth. Take as much care in buying your supplements as you do your food. Talk to a naturopathic doctor, dietitian, nutritionist, or knowledgeable supplements retailer for more insight and recommendations.

THREE KEY SUPPLEMENTS FOR THREE KEY PHASES

Diet and lifestyle factors are the foundation of any woman's wellness program, but dietary supplementation also can complement a health plan. To simplify supplementation for my patients, I have created a three-stage program that features three key products appropriate for each life stage.

The three key products I recommend are
1. quality multivitamin/mineral formula to support overall health,
2. bone-health formula to keep bones strong, and
3. A hormone balancer containing herbs and nutrients appropriate for each life stage to support healthy hormone function.

Phase One—Estrogen levels are high and overall hormonal activity is fairly stable. The time between puberty and mid-30s is typically characterized as phase one and is an ideal time to establish bone health and consistent hormone balance for a lifetime. During this time, every woman should take a daily multivitamin and mineral formula that provides antioxidants and vitamins D and K. Because there's not enough calcium in a multivitamin, an additional calcium and phosphorus supplement will help maintain optimum bone health. Finally, women should also look for a hormone-balancing supplement to help neutralize mood swings, PMS, and menstrual cramps and to help keep weight optimal and fatigue at bay. This type of supplement is likely to include DIM, phosphatidylcholine, and vitamin E.

Phase Two—During the perimenopausal years, estrogen levels can become erratic, causing insomnia, fatigue, irregular periods, and mood swings. This phase is beginning earlier than ever before and can start when a woman is in her 30s. I believe women need increased hormonal support and bone nutrients at this time. Again, I recommend a comprehensive multivitamin and mineral supplement in addition to a bone-health supplement designed to maintain bone health in women during their perimenopausal years. The third component for women in phase two is a supplement or combination of supplements for any symptoms of perimenopause they might be experiencing. Black cohosh (*Cimicifuga racemosa*) for hot flashes, night sweats, and mood swings; green tea for energy and weight management; chaste tree berry (*Vitex agnus-castus*) for menstrual symptoms; rhodiola (*Rhodiola rosea*) for concentration and mental alertness; and valerian (*Valeriana officinalis*), hops (*Humulus lupulus*), and L-theanine for relaxation and sleep quality. (Detailed information on these and other natural remedies for symptom relief is available in Chapter 7.)

Phase Three—Menstruation stops when hormone levels drop to trigger the onset of menopause. To help alleviate menopausal symptoms, women need specific herbs and nutrients. They also need extra bone-building vitamins and minerals. The age of menopause is typically 51 but can vary. For women in this phase, the multivitamin and mineral formula I recommend contains antioxidants plus lutein and soy. Lutein supports eye health, and soy helps with menopausal symptoms, heart health, bone health, and cancer prevention. The bone-support supplement from phase two is still appropriate here. The third component for phase three is again similar to phase two, but women might also choose to look for something with ginseng (*Panax* spp) for additional energy.

By adjusting the three key components for each stage, the supplement program I recommend provides at least a minimum comprehensive supply of vitamins, minerals, nutrients, and herbs to support a woman through all the stages of her life.

ACTIVITY IS THE ANSWER

The next element of a strong foundation is exercise. I have yet to find a more powerful health tool. Even though we all know physical activity is a major component of good health, only 20 percent of Americans exercise regularly. The good news is once you start to exercise, the benefits will help you stick with it for a lifetime. With physical activity the body becomes stronger, has enhanced endurance, and functions more efficiently. Truly, the entire body benefits from the enhanced cardiovascular and respiratory function. This means more oxygen goes to your cells, and more carbon dioxide goes out of your body. And the health rewards of consistent physical activity go far beyond maintaining a healthy weight, even though that's important. Results of scientific studies have shown that exercise can stimulate a positive immune response, enhance heart health, and improve mood and self-image.

Beginning an exercise program may not be easy, but it is critical to your overall health and your ability to relieve the symptoms of hormone imbalance. Exercise promotes lean body mass, burns fat, and aids digestion and elimination; these qualities help keep hormones in balance. Among its many other benefits, exercise also improves bone density and sleep quality, eases hot flashes, reduces anxiety and stress, and enhances brain function.

In a report featured in *Sports Medicine,* researchers concluded that strength training helps prevent osteoporosis, increase energy levels, normalize blood pressure and blood sugar, and decrease body fat. Studies indicate inactive people gain excess fat and lose up to 10 percent of their muscle mass each decade after age 30. Increased fat and reduced muscle mass is a dangerous combination. That's why it's especially important to include strength training in your weekly routine. Strength training, including sit-ups, push-ups, and weight lifting, increases bone density and muscle mass while speeding up metabolism. According to Edward Laskowski, MD, codirector of the Sports Medicine Center at Mayo Clinic, you can see dramatic improvements with only 20 minutes of strength training two to three times a week.

RE-CREATE WITH RECREATION

Being active is fun. Not only is it a way for us to nurture ourselves, it provides a social outlet. I like to think of recreation as "re-creation." Physical activity is a way for us to re-create and re-capture vitality. Here are a few helpful hints for your exercise routine.

Consistency is more important than intensity. Doing something physical every day for at least 30 minutes will provide more benefit than waiting until Friday and going for a four-hour hike or playing tennis for two hours.

Stretch! This is especially important for older women. Every time you are involved in physical activity, you should stretch your muscles after they are warmed up. Yoga, qi gong, pilates, or other stretching-based exercise programs are great options.

Create fitness goals. Remember to increase your level of intensity the more physically fit you become.

Share the experience. Some of my patients tell me it helps to exercise with a friend. Find a buddy who will try a new class with you or walk with you at some time during the day. When exercise has a social element, it is more fun and you won't want to miss it. For some, it helps to verbalize exercise goals to supportive family and friends. Once you've made your commitment out loud, you're less likely to neglect your program.

NEW WAYS TO MOVE

Bored with the gym? Try these ideas to spice up your exercise routine.

- Take a dance class (ballroom, swing, jazz, salsa, hip hop, country western line or square dancing, and belly dancing are just a few ideas).
- Learn a new sport (maybe golf, tennis, or racquetball).
- Try a new class (have you taken yoga, tai chi, qi gong, kick boxing, NIA, or pilates?).
- Walk (pedometers are an inexpensive way to quantify your movement and to get you to take more steps every day).

A new form of exercise can invigorate you and renew your motivation to a fitness routine. And the more you like what you're doing, the more likely you are to keep doing it.

If you have been sedentary for years or if you have a history of heart disease or other serious illness, get some guidance regarding the appropriate exercise program for you. Talk to a healthcare provider and a personal trainer to create a workout you like and that works for you. My exercise philosophy is to make it fun. Find something you enjoy doing (gardening, biking, swimming, tennis, dancing, golfing) or some new activity, and then incorporate it into your weekly routine. If exercise is fun, you will look forward to it and be more apt to keep those exercise appointments in your busy schedule. A good goal is to exercise for 30 minutes a day three days a week and gradually make it a daily ritual.

THE MIND/BODY/EMOTION CONNECTION

In addition to good food, appropriate supplements, and daily exercise, a healthy mental outlook further strengthens your foundation. Don't overlook the critical connection between mind and body. What affects our emotions affects us on a cellular level. Issues such as stress, hostility, isolation, unresolved emotional issues, and sadness can negatively affect our health. Conversely, love, humor, and support can contribute to our healing.

In several recent studies, researchers have demonstrated that support from loving friends and family positively influences immune system health. One study, featured in *JAMA*, indicated women with previous chest pain or who had had a heart attack were almost three times more likely to have a second heart problem if they had marital stress. The roles of a supportive partner or network of friends and family cannot be underestimated in well-being and a healthy lifestyle.

Another contributor to mind/body/emotion well-being is laughter. Don't belittle the power of this healing tool. When was the last time you had a hearty belly laugh? If you pause for too long before answering, chances are you need more humor in your life. A study featured in *Oncology Nursing Forum* confirmed humor helps cancer patients cope with their illness. If you haven't had the giggles in a long time, consider a night out at a local comedy club; rent a weekend full of the silliest comedies you can find; have a pillow fight with children, grandchildren, or your partner; read a funny book—just find something to help you lighten up and laugh.

Psychotherapy can also be a helpful tool for resolving past issues or present conflicts in a safe environment. I have personally found psychotherapy to be a powerful resource on my journey toward healing and health. The biggest misconception out there is that psychotherapy is only for the mentally ill, for crisis management, or for people dealing with traumatic issues. In reality, developing a therapeutic relationship with a qualified professional can provide the safety and containment we not only need, but—on a deeper level—I believe we crave. This type of processing helps us go deeper into awareness of ourselves and how we relate to the world in which we exist. The healing power of this intimate understanding of ourselves cannot be measured.

BUILD YOUR FOUNDATION FIRST

By concentrating on factors we can control, such as diet, lifestyle habits, dietary supplementation, and emotional well-being, we can build a solid health foundation that will help us heal from illness and keep us well. Focus on building a strong foundation first. After the foundation is in place, the framework of any comprehensive wellness program begins with healthy digestion.

CHAPTER 4

Proper Digestion is Critical

Most people don't think about how important good digestion is to hormone balance and overall health. But the fact is the digestive system is imperative to both these issues and works closely with the endocrine system. Hormones help direct digestion, and proper digestion positively influences hormonal activity. Conversely, poor digestion, specifically a sluggish liver, can contribute to hormone imbalance. If the feedback loop that manages digestion is not functioning properly, the effects may begin with an upset stomach or constipation, but they will eventually reach far beyond. To help you keep your digestive system working properly, it helps to understand its basic mechanics.

THE DIGESTIVE SYSTEM

What is proper digestion? At its simplest, it is food processing. The digestive system breaks down, assimilates, and absorbs nutrients from the things we eat and drink. Digestion involves complex mechanical and chemical operations to ensure your body is properly fueled and rid of waste products. From end to end, your entire digestive system measures about 30 feet. The key organs of this expansive system include the oral cavity (teeth, tongue, salivary glands), the esophagus, stomach, liver, gallbladder, pancreas, small intestine, large intestine (colon), and the rectum. Here is an overview of how the digestive system works.

1. You take a bite of food and begin to chew. The material is mechanically macerated and mixed with saliva, which contains enzymes that begin breaking food down and preparing it for the next digestive step. This process also signals other parts of the system to prepare for incoming food. Unfortunately, we often rush this vital first step. To give digestion a good head start, chew foods thoroughly.

2. In the stomach, your meal is further broken down with chemical secretions and churning action. The stomach produces numerous secretions, including hydrochloric acid and pepsin, which facilitate proper digestion and absorption.
3. Food moves through the digestive system via rhythmic contractions of your intestinal muscles, called peristalsis, which push the food from one part to the next.
4. The small intestines absorb nutrients, which pass through the lining and into the bloodstream or lymph fluids. The absorbed nutrients are metabolized and used by every cell, organ, and system in the body.
5. The gallbladder, pancreas, and liver all produce enzymes and other secretions that assist food breakdown and absorption. For example, the pancreas produces proteases that help digest protein. The liver manufactures bile, which aids in absorbing fats, oils, and fat-soluble vitamins.
6. The end of the line is the five-foot colon, which absorbs water, electrolytes, and any final useful byproducts of digestion. Indigestible food particles, bacteria, and toxins that have no use or are harmful are eliminated from the body.

Digestion couldn't happen without the endocrine system, which produces hormones that control the necessary chemical activities. Hormones influence the type, amount, and timing of digestive chemicals released. For example, endocrine system hormones stimulate enzyme activity and adjust sugar metabolism in the liver. When the endocrine system is functioning properly, the digestive system can do its job efficiently. Effective digestion results in absorption of nutrients necessary for optimal endocrine function. It is all connected.

If one system is not working properly, the other is affected. That's why heartburn or constipation, for example, combined with fatigue, irritability, loss of libido, or foggy thinking, can be linked to an underlying hormone imbalance. Taking antacids or laxatives may help digestion-related symptoms but will not address the underlying cause. In addition, simply masking symptoms creates an unhealthy cycle of dependence on expensive medications that do nothing to effect a cure. Plus, these drugs are not benign.

THE PROBLEM WITH ANTACIDS

Antacids are a $3 billion a year business. Antacid producers want you to believe their symptom-relief product is the best route to take for digestive upsets, but there are several reasons to think twice before you plop-plop-fizz-fizz or "purple pill" your way to relief. These products alter stomach acidity, mineral status, and body pH, as well as compromise the immune system.

In the short-term, antacids neutralize stomach acids and provide relief of heartburn and indigestion. However, stomach acids are necessary for food digestion and vitamin absorption. Tinkering with acid production long-term can adversely affect health. And antacids do nothing to heal an inflamed or injured stomach lining.

A German researcher reports antacids have also been shown to deplete calcium and phosphorus, which weakens bones; promote alkalosis, which can harm the kidneys and heart; trigger gastric acid secretion, which can cause kidney stones; and damage the lining of the esophagus, which can lead to cancer. Additionally, the immune system is compromised, because blocking hydrochloric acid production encourages overgrowth of harmful bacteria and toxins.

Common digestive problems are not caused by excess acid production. The body produces stomach acid because it is needed to digest foods. Many digestive problems are a result of poor food and lifestyle choices. A diet rich in fresh fruits and vegetables, which contain natural enzymes, is important to healthy digestion and, in the long run, will be far more beneficial than an antacid.

Although hormone imbalance can cause digestive problems, it is more common for digestive problems to cause hormone imbalance. Various factors contribute.

• A diet rich in saturated fat, chemicals, additives, simple sugars, red meat, artificial sweeteners, and refined carbohydrates does not contain the enzymes important for digestive processes and can lead to destruction of good bacteria and an overgrowth of harmful bacteria in the gastrointestinal tract.

• Not eating enough fiber-rich foods leads to poor elimination and therefore poor detoxification. Fiber is critical for the removal of indigestible substances and harmful bacteria, parasites, and other toxins that can come from foods. When these toxins aren't eliminated, the liver becomes overburdened by the accumulation. Symptoms such as chronic fatigue, headaches, and autoimmune diseases can manifest. The overburdened liver is also less able to metabolize hormones, leading to imbalance.

• Dehydration interferes with proper digestion, because water is critical to the process.

• Prescription and over-the-counter medications, such as birth control pills, HRT, antibiotics, antacids, and nonsteroidal anti-inflammatory drugs (NSAIDs), disrupt digestion in numerous ways, including increasing overgrowth of harmful bacteria and increasing acidity, which can deteriorate the stomach lining.

In addition to these dietary factors, the two biggest digestive problems that disrupt hormonal balance are bacterial imbalance and leaky gut syndrome.

BACTERIAL TURF WARS

Bacteria are everywhere. There are more bacteria in and on you than there are people on this planet. About one trillion bacteria live in your intestines alone. Both beneficial and harmful bacteria move and adapt at an amazing pace. As they fight for internal turf control, their objective is to secure positions along the digestive tract so they can stick, multiply, and colonize.

Proper bacterial balance benefits digestive health and therefore overall health. There are internal and external sources of both harmful and beneficial bacteria. The digestive system is designed to produce beneficial bacteria to keep the population of harmful bacteria in check. Your health depends on the beneficial bacteria prevailing.

One way to increase your numbers of beneficial bacteria is to take a probiotic dietary supplement. It is important to find a probiotic with a delivery system that ensures protection against stomach acid so the bacteria can be delivered to the intestines. The two key beneficial bacteria are acidophilus (*Lactobacillus acidophilus*) and bifidus (*Bifidobacterium longum*). Acidophilus primarily focuses on the small intestines; bifidus works in the large intestines. Together they produce substances that deactivate the harmful bacteria, change the acidity of the internal environment so the harmful bacteria can't thrive, deprive harmful bacteria of nutrients so they can't survive, and produce an antibioticlike substance that kills the harmful bacteria.

Sometimes, because of our lifestyle and dietary choices, the bad guys gain an advantage. Certain circumstances encourage harmful bacterial overgrowth, including the following.

• **Prescription drugs.** Antibiotics, birth control pills, and HRT can kill beneficial as well as harmful bacteria, disrupting internal ecology.

• **Food and water contaminants.** The foods we eat and the water we drink can contain parasites and harmful bacteria that wreak havoc on our internal bacterial balance.

• **Travel.** The chances of acquiring a parasite or bacteria from food or water increases when we travel, especially abroad.

• **Diet and lifestyle.** A low-fiber diet, increased alcohol consumption, lack of physical activity, smoking, and increased emotional or physical stress can cause harmful bacteria populations to surge.

When harmful bacteria take over, they can damage the intestinal lining and leak out into the rest of the body. When the intestinal lining becomes permeable, a condition called leaky gut syndrome develops.

LEAKY GUT

When the wrong kind of bacteria populate the small intestine, their activities produce compounds that constrict and relax blood vessels. Too much of this causes spaces to develop between the cells of the intestinal lining. Spaces allow bacteria, toxins, and large food particles to seep into the bloodstream and circulate throughout the body. It is problematic that food is not being broken down properly and vital nutrients are not being absorbed, and that harmful bacteria and toxins are not being eliminated. When this occurs, virtually any system in the body can be negatively affected, resulting in a broad range of symptoms and potential illnesses ranging from diarrhea to arthritis.

When the gut leaks these foreign, larger molecules into the bloodstream, the immune system identifies them as dangerous and moves into action. The immune system, which is designed to identify and kill harmful invaders, becomes strained as it tries to keep up. In addition to stressing the immune system, leaky gut negatively affects the liver, which is taxed trying to eliminate these excess toxins. As a result, the liver can become weak and unable to detoxify excess hormones, which can contribute to an imbalance.

Eating a healthy, balanced diet will help prevent leaky gut syndrome. In addition, recognizing digestive problems early and supporting them with natural alternatives is important to preventing problems such as leaky gut syndrome, as well as bacterial and hormonal imbalances.

NATURAL DIGESTIVE AIDS

According to the National Institutes of Health (NIH), 60 million to 70 million people have digestive disorders, accounting for 50 million physician office visits each year. Some 10 percent of Americans experience heartburn every day, and 44 percent feel the burn at least monthly, according to the American Academy of Family Physicians. All of this discomfort sends people searching for relief. More than 25 million Americans opt for antacids at least twice a week. Often they're lured by the ubiquitous ads for Zantac, Pepcid, and Prilosec, but there are gentler remedies that work with the body instead of against it.

I recognize my patients' need for symptom relief, but I believe in helping them understand the underlying causes of their digestive discomfort. Often, I recommend dietary supplements in addition to diet and lifestyle advice to help ease the uncomfortable symptoms associated with digestive disturbances. Following are some examples, but please speak with your healthcare provider before taking any dietary supplement.

For peptic ulcers, deglycyrrhizinated licorice (DGL) is great. This form of licorice has the portion of the herb that can cause serious side effects, such as hypertension, removed. Commission E, Germany's equivalent to the FDA, approved DGL as an ulcer treatment. Results of several comparison studies show DGL is more effective than the drug Tagamet at healing ulcers and preventing recurrence. DGL works by protecting and healing the stomach lining, not by blocking the production of stomach acid, which interferes with proper digestion. An effective dose of DGL must be chewed, because mixing with saliva stimulates its activity.

Irritable bowel syndrome (IBS) symptoms can be treated with enteric-coated peppermint oil or artichoke leaf. Both these herbs have been shown to help with IBS-associated cramping, pain, bloating, gas, and constipation. In a case study published in *Alternative Medicine Review,* a patient taking enteric-coated peppermint oil experienced improvement in IBS symptoms. In a clinical trial, enteric-coated peppermint oil reduced the severity of IBS pain in

75 percent of the children who received it. Artichoke leaf extract proved useful in a group of IBS patients; they reported significant reductions in symptom severity and favorably rated its effectiveness. Researchers whose work was published in *Phytotherapy Research* concluded the results support the notion that artichoke leaf extract may be valuable for relieving IBS symptoms.

For gas, bloating, and constipation not associated with IBS or for heartburn, digestive enzymes taken with meals can help. Dietary enzymes encourage balanced enzyme activity, which improves digestion. I recommend a blend of enzymes that help break down carbohydrates, proteins, and fats. Look for a product containing amylase, protease, lipase, lactase, phytase, cellulase, sucrase, and maltase. The bacteria acidophilus and bifidus also produce natural enzymes that not only help keep harmful bacteria at bay, but encourage healthy digestion as well.

DIGESTIVE RELIEF AT A GLANCE

Complaint	Remedy	Dose
Constipation	Fiber	25-30 g/day (sources include food, bran, psyllium, and flaxseed)
	Water	Eight 8-oz glasses/day
IBS	Enteric-coated peppermint oil	0.2 mL 3 times/day between meals
	Artichoke leaf (*Cynara scolymus*)	1 teaspoon liquid extract mixed with water, a 320-mg standardized extract capsule, or 15–30 drops tincture mixed into water three times/day
Indigestion, heartburn	Artichoke leaf (*Cynara scolymus*)	1 teaspoon liquid extract mixed with water, a 320-mg standardized extract capsule, or 15–30 drops tincture mixed into water three times/day
	Ginger (*Zingiber officinale*)	100 mg/day of a product standardized to contain 20 percent gingerol active oils
	Greater celandine (*Chelidonium majus*)	4 mg standardized extract 3 times/day or 1–3 ml tincture in water before meals
	Enzymes	Take digestive enzymes before meals; follow product instructions
Peptic ulcers	DGL	Chew 2–3 380-mg tablets before meals and bedtime, or follow product instructions

Raw, unprocessed foods contain enzymes that assist digestion, so eating more of these will encourage healthy enzyme activity. Add more fresh fruits and vegetables, especially garlic, cabbage, and red peppers, to your diet to maintain healthy enzymatic activity and therefore healthy digestion.

In addition to supporting your digestive processes, which in turn supports hormone balance, it is important to tend to your liver. This organ bears the brunt of the body's detoxification duties, and detoxification is a key part of digestion and hormone balance.

LOVE YOUR LIVER

When it comes to healthy digestion and efficient detoxification of toxins and excess estrogens, it is all about liver function. The liver performs more than 500 physiologic functions. To keep this large glandular organ operating at its peak requires some special care. I recommend a dietary supplement with liver-supporting herbs and nutrients, and also a periodic cleanse.

Liver support—The most widely studied herb for liver health is **milk thistle** (*Silybum marianum*). This herb's active constituent is silymarin and is typically standardized at 80 percent. The German Commission E approved an oral extract for treating liver disease in 1986. Milk thistle is said to work by displacing toxins trying to bind to the liver as well as spurring liver regeneration. This herb is widely used to treat alcoholic hepatitis, alcoholic fatty liver, liver cirrhosis, liver poisoning, and viral hepatitis. In a study published in the *Journal of Hepatology,* researchers reported treating cirrhosis patients with milk thistle was effective, and survival rates increased.

Dandelion root (*Taraxacum officinale*) supports healthy bile flow from the gallbladder, which promotes digestion and makes the liver's job easier. In a study published in the *International Journal of Clinical Chemistry,* researchers conducting an animal study found dandelion extract improved fat metabolism in diabetic rats. Human trials are necessary to further determine benefit, but based on historical uses, dandelion is likely a useful liver-support herb. Dandelion is also a mild bitter, which means it stimulates secretion of digestive juices in the stomach, aiding digestion. The Commission E has approved dandelion root extract for indigestion, to stimulate appetite, and as a diuretic.

Artichoke leaf (*Cynara scolymus*) is also an approved treatment in Europe for indigestion. In addition to stimulating healthy bile production,

A CAST OF LIVER SUPPORTERS

Supplement	Dose
Artichoke	40 mg/day
Dandelion	10 mg/day
Milk thistle	100 mg/day
SAMe	Dose varies depending on the support needed; however, SAMe has been shown to be safe and effective at doses between 200 and 1,200 mg daily.

several clinical studies indicate artichoke leaf extract supports overall gastrointestinal function. A researcher reporting in *Planta Medica* states the results of a study involving water-soluble artichoke extracts indicate this herb has potent bile-stimulating properties, which may contribute to its ability to protect the liver. Artichoke leaf should be standardized at 13 percent to 18 percent of caffeoylquinic acids, which are the active compounds.

The dietary supplement **SAMe** (S-adenosylmethionine) has shown promise in cases of liver disease. SAMe is a natural methyl donor, meaning it is a molecule made in the body that gives part of itself to other molecules so they can function properly. When combined with folic acid and vitamin B12, SAMe makes a contribution to nearly every bodily function. By producing the extremely powerful antioxidant glutathione, which enhances the liver's ability to clear out toxins, SAMe promotes efficient liver function. Research indicates SAMe may benefit livers impaired by alcohol-induced cirrhosis, drug toxicity, hepatitis, and cholestasis. In a review of studies conducted with SAMe, researchers concluded the supplement counteracts the effects of liver toxins by promoting bile secretion. Further, they say both intravenous and oral doses of SAMe significantly improve bile function. According to results of numerous trials, SAMe is an effective and safe way to manage liver conditions. Because SAMe is a highly reactive molecule, this supplement must be enteric-coated and taken on an empty stomach.

Cleanse—A great way to support liver function is with a regular, comprehensive, gentle cleanse or detoxification. I liken it to changing my car's oil every 3,000 miles. Because of the toxins we encounter in our modern lives, we need to take the same kind of preventive care of our bodies as we do our cars. I recommend a 10- to 14-day cleanse program four times a year. Doing a cleanse at the beginning of each season is a good way to remember. The cleanse includes liver support, which is critical because of the liver's significant role in detoxification. There are three components:

1. A cleansing laxative formula that promotes healthy bowel elimination. The one I like includes an herbal mucilage blend [slippery elm (*Ulmus rubra*), marshmallow (*Althaea officinalis*), and fenugreek (*Trigonella foenum-graecum*)], an herbal soothing blend [peppermint (*Mentha x piperita*), fennel (*Foeniculum vulgare*), and ginger (*Zingiber officinale*)], burdock (*Arctium lappa*), and red clover (*Trifolium pratense*).

2. A fiber formula that binds to the toxins the laxative formula has loosened and helps to improve colon function. Look for one with ingredients including psyllium (*Plantago ovata*), oat (*Avena sativa*), guar gum (*Cyamopsis tetragonoloba*), pectin (from citrus fruit), and marshmallow (*Althaea officinalis*).

3. The herbs milk thistle, artichoke, licorice, and dandelion to support optimal liver function and assist detoxification.

Talk to your healthcare provider about a customized liver-support program. A naturopathic doctor or other healthcare provider can help you find a cleanse program right for you.

SUPPORT YOUR SYSTEMS

We have an incredible internal system that helps us optimize the benefits of the foods we eat by supporting the body's functions and eliminating waste. Supporting and enhancing digestion is extremely important to maintaining or gaining hormonal balance and for overall health. But there are other things that can negatively affect our ability to keep a healthy balance. One all-too-common culprit is stress. Stress caused by today's fast-paced world challenges our ability to stay healthy. Controlling stress and supporting our bodies during difficult times is important, because the physiologic effects of stress are far-reaching. If we are to ease symptoms and prevent serious illness, it is important to understand the stress connection.

CHAPTER 5

The Stress Connection

Stress is nearly impossible to avoid. Economic uncertainties and world-wide problems compound the hectic pace of our daily lives. Many of my patients feel overwhelmed, anxious, and depressed on a regular basis. But stress is a normal experience, and our reaction to stress is necessary for survival. The stress response gets us to work on time, helps us meet important deadlines, and gets us out of the way of a moving car. Our bodies are designed to handle stress by way of an internal defense mechanism known as the fight-or-flight response. Chronic, unrelenting stress, however, has a devastating effect on the body.

Centuries ago, people were often faced with life-threatening stressors, quite different from the ones we routinely experience today. Even though we are no longer battling wild animals or other attackers, our bodies respond to the perceived stress the same way. Whether we are running from a burning building or to work because we are late, the internal reaction is identical. To narrowly escape a car accident, for example, the hypothalamus sends a message to the adrenal gland telling it to release the hormones adrenaline and noradrenaline. These hormones circulate and influence other glands and systems. Heart rate increases. Bronchioles in the lungs dilate to make breathing more efficient. The pancreas pours more glucose into the bloodstream in case we need more energy. Digestive activity decreases to conserve energy. Muscles tense, blood sugar levels rise, and there is an increased tendency for blood to clot. This is the body's way of preparing to fight or flee and cope with the consequences of either decision.

This physiological reaction is normal and necessary. But stress becomes dangerous when it feels like we are constantly being chased. This excessive, unrelenting stress actually causes us to develop a sort of "panic biochemistry," because we are on a continuous heightened state of alert. The results can be overwhelming and harmful.

A WOMAN'S RESPONSE TO STRESS

Results of a study published in *Psychological Review* in 2000 suggest women may respond to stress differently than men. Instead of fight or flee, women can tend or befriend in the face of stress. Researchers found when the hormone oxytocin is released as part of a woman's stress response, it tempers the fight-or-flight instinct and urges her to tend children and be with other women. When she opts for tending and befriending, it seems more oxytocin is released, producing a calming effect.

The calming response doesn't occur in men, though, because testosterone reduces the effects of oxytocin. According to the researchers, estrogen enhances it. The researchers theorize the tend-or-befriend response helps women consistently outlive men.

Whatever you do, don't neglect your girlfriends when you're stressed—they're good for your health. Friendships have actually been shown to improve health and help us live longer. People without friends were more likely to die in a six-month period than those who had close relationships, according to results of one study. In another, researchers found people with the most friends cut their risk of dying by 60 percent in a nine-year period. And Nurses' Health Study researchers concluded the more friends a woman has, the less likely she is to develop physical impairments as she ages. The results were significant enough that researchers concluded not having close friends is as damaging to your health as smoking or being overweight.

THE ROAD TO IMBALANCE

The internal control mechanisms associated with stress are known as the sympathetic and parasympathetic nervous systems. These two systems balance each other to help us cope with stress consistently. When you are awake, you are operating mostly in the sympathetic mode as you multitask your way through the day. Your adrenal glands (your stress glands) are most active during this time, helping your body adapt to whatever challenges and tasks you face. The parasympathetic mode is primarily in charge at night, when the body rests, relaxes, and repairs. This time in parasympathetic mode is critical. As long as your body has time to calm down after an intense moment or day, your health will not be negatively affected.

Problems arise, however, when we stay in the sympathetic mode too long. Overwork, insomnia, stimulants such as caffeine, junk foods, and lack of exercise can all hinder parasympathetic function. When we don't relax, rest, and recharge, we get tired, which starts a vicious cycle. When we're tired, we tend not to exercise, we use more stimulants, and we make unhealthy dietary choices such as high-carbohydrate convenience foods, all of which further stress the adrenal glands that are already working overtime dealing with unrelenting stress.

To cope with increasing stress levels, the adrenal glands, which contain two major parts, the medulla and the cortex, secrete hormones. In response to stress perceived by the brain, the medulla secretes epinephrine and norepinephrine (these hormones are called catecholamines). These chemicals help the body respond to stress by increasing heart rate, blood pressure, breath rate, blood sugar levels, and cellular metabolism. The cortex produces a wide range of chemicals, including cortisol (glucocorticoid) and aldosterone (mineralocorticoid). These hormones regulate inflammation responses, immune function, mineral balance, and metabolic and reproductive function. Cortisol is our main stress-response hormone. These necessary energy and circulatory adaptations, combined with the other changes the adrenals stimulate in the body during times of stress, can—if stressful periods are prolonged—increase the risk of exhaustion and various disease states.

If the stress continues and the adrenals keep to their increased cortisol-production rate, your body can convert progesterone, one of the sex hormones, into cortisol if needed. The body is designed to choose survival over reproduction and will sacrifice progesterone, a key reproductive hormone, in an effort to survive. To the body, prolonged stress is the same, whether you are being chased by wild animals or worrying about bills or the health of a loved one. It will do whatever it takes to survive the attack, even if it means losing valuable progesterone. The resulting progesterone deficiency can lead to estrogen dominance.

In addition to depleting progesterone, increased cortisol levels caused by stress can leech calcium from bones, making them more fragile and prone to fracture. High cortisol levels also stimulate appetite. Many of my patients report that when they are under continual, intense stress, they eat more and typically crave unhealthy foods. This perpetuates a vicious cycle of unhealthy behavior. Excess cortisol production is also linked to increased abdominal fat, which creates the "apple-shaped" figure (meaning fat deposits in the middle) that has been linked to increased risk of heart disease, diabetes, and cancer.

Cortisol isn't the only hormone affected by adrenal overwork. In addition to stress hormones, the adrenal glands secrete pregnenolone, DHEA, testosterone, progesterone, and estrogen. If the body is trying desperately to cope with stress, the adrenal glands are unable to secrete the hormones necessary to carry out other bodily functions. When one gland or system in the body is weak or sluggish, it affects other systems—especially the heart, blood vessels, and immune system—until all internal systems are so bogged down that you can't function properly.

According to author and clinician Jesse Lynn Hanley, MD, if we do not allow our adrenal glands to rest and repair, we are sure to become victims of adrenal burnout. In Hanley's book on the subject, *Tired of Being Tired* (Putnam Pub Group, 2001), she says adrenal burnout is serious and can cause anxiety, autoimmune diseases, chronic fatigue, depression, migraines, type-2 diabetes, infertility, heart disease, sore muscles, and weight gain or loss.

HABITS THAT LEAD TO ADRENAL BURNOUT

According to Jesse Lynn Hanley, MD, author of *Tired of Being Tired*, the following characteristics and habits describe the ideal candidate for adrenal burnout.

- Skipping meals/dieting
- Eating processed or junk foods
- Exercising too little or too much
- Worrying and not making time for relaxation and fun
- Not getting enough sleep or ignoring fatigue to finish the day's work
- Using stimulants such as sugar, caffeine, nicotine, drugs, and certain herbs to increase function when tired
- Breathing shallowly when tense
- Exposure to environmental toxins (household products and food)
- Putting yourself last

How many of these characteristics describe you? How much downtime do you give yourself each day? Are you allowing your body to relax and repair?

In my clinical practice, I find that patients who experience continual, intense stress have weak adrenal gland function. Not surprisingly, these women also have symptoms of overall hormonal imbalance that can include PMS, hot flashes, night sweats, insomnia, and diminished libido. When we address adrenal fatigue, the women's symptoms are eased and they have more energy and vitality.

Our adrenal glands are the built-in backup system for postmenopause hormone production. They are meant to step up to the plate when our ovaries take their well-deserved break. If a woman in transition to menopause has a difficult time, which we have seen increasingly in the last several decades, the first thing to address is her adrenals. It is about restoring function, not replacing it.

SUPPORTING ADRENAL FUNCTION

Our adrenal glands are the front-line defense against stress-related symptoms and illnesses. In addition, their proper function is critical to overall health and hormone balance. The best way to support adrenal gland function is to rest. You must make time to allow your parasympathetic mode to work its magic. During rest, internal systems repair and restore balance disrupted during the sympathetic, hectic pace of the day. Another way to support adrenal health is with a sensible whole-foods diet and prudent supplementation.

Certain specific herbs and nutrients can help support healthy adrenal function. Vitamin C, ginseng (*Panax* spp), and rhodiola (*Rhodiola rosea*) have all been shown to provide powerful, natural support during stressful times.

Vitamin C is an important antioxidant involved in numerous biochemical reactions that positively influence overall health. In addition to nourishing the adrenal glands, vitamin C enhances heart, immune, and detoxification function. In a double-blind, placebo-controlled trial conducted in Germany, researchers found that 3 grams of vitamin C in divided, sustained-release doses kept blood pressure, anxiety, and cortisol production under control after a stressful situation. The work, published in *Psychopharmacology,* indicates high doses of vitamin C can mediate the physiological effects of stress. Although vitamin C is an ingredient in most quality multivitamins, you may need a higher dose during times of stress. Work with a qualified healthcare professional to determine how much, if any, extra vitamin C you need.

Chinese ginseng (*Panax ginseng*) and Siberian ginseng (*Eleutherococcus senticosus*) are considered adaptogenic herbs. An adaptogen is a substance with a normalizing and restorative effect; it can improve your resistance to stress. The ginsengs help restore balance and promote overall well-being. Ginseng also is frequently referred to as an adrenal tonic, because it increases the tone and function of the adrenal glands. In a double-blind clinical trial, researchers evaluated the effect of ginseng on nurses who had switched from day to night duty. The nurses rated themselves on baseline competence, well-being, and mood and were tested for performance and blood chemistry. After the trial, the group taking Chinese ginseng scored higher compared with the placebo group when they were remeasured. Ginseng made the nurses feel more alert yet tranquil and better able to perform their jobs.

In other work, South Korean researchers concluded ginseng is useful for treating stress-related disorders. Based on the animal and human research, ginseng is beneficial for people with stress and anxiety. How should you choose your ginseng? Chinese ginseng is more potent than Siberian ginseng, so for substantial stress and adrenal dysfunction, the former is the best choice. For mild to moderate stress, Siberian ginseng is a wise starting point.

Rhodiola has been used for centuries in Eastern Europe and Asia to stimulate the nervous system, decrease depression, enhance work performance, eliminate fatigue, and prevent high-altitude sickness. Russian researchers also have found rhodiola can increase resistance to various chemical, biological, and physical stressors. The *Alternative Medicine Review* reported rhodiola can relieve symptoms associated with intense physical or intellectual strain, including sleep difficulties, poor appetite, irritability, hypertension, headaches, and fatigue.

Several studies have demonstrated rhodiola is an effective antifatigue agent. Russian researchers combined rhodiola with ginseng and found the combination positively influenced brain function after sleep deprivation. The journal *Phytomedicine* featured a study involving 56 young, healthy, night-duty physicians who took rhodiola and found the herb reduced fatigue under stressful conditions.

THE THYROID LINK

In addition to supporting adrenal function, maintaining thyroid health is important for controlling the effects of the stress response. The thyroid gland is affected by stress and intimately connected to adrenal function. When the adrenals are overstressed, the thyroid gland works harder in an attempt to compensate and will eventually succumb to the overwork. The thyroid serves many important functions, including controlling metabolism, heart rate, and bone health. Unrelenting stress causes the body to make compromises.

The thyroid gland is also the body's internal thermostat; it regulates body temperature by secreting two hormones that control how quickly the body burns calories and uses energy. Enzymes that run every system and process in your body depend on the thyroid to keep the internal temperature at 98.6 degrees F. If body temperature is much lower, the enzymes can't function properly, causing the body to operate inefficiently. During stressful times the body conserves energy. Sometimes this means lowering body temperature temporarily. After the stress has passed, the body restores the temperature to normal, and the systems return to their optimal functioning status. After repeated or sustained episodes of stress, it becomes more difficult to return to normal. In time, when the thyroid gland realizes the stress is not ending, it slows down to conserve energy.

The thyroid takes direction from the pituitary gland, which is stimulated by the hypothalamus. If the thyroid gland is weak, is not functioning properly, or is not getting enough iodine or L-tyrosine—the building block of thyroid hormones—from a healthy diet, it cannot make the hormones necessary to perform its duties. As a result of the pituitary's prompting, the thyroid gland grows in a vain attempt to produce more hormones. This enlargement is medically known as a goiter and can be caused by hypofunction (decreased function) or hyperfunction (increased function).

Hypothyroidism occurs when the thyroid does not produce enough hormones. This condition is more common than hyperthyroidism and is characterized by weight gain, hair loss, constipation, cold hands and feet, exhaustion, joint aches, and a slow heart rate. Estimates indicate more than 11 million Americans have some degree of hypothyroidism. However, many cases are misdiagnosed or go undetected because of limitations with present testing methods.

TESTING THYROID FUNCTION

There is some controversy about the best way to test thyroid function. Conventional medicine relies on a blood test to measure circulating thyroid and pituitary hormones. This test, however, can't always determine if there is a problem. In many cases, even though a person has many of the clinical symptoms of hypothyroidism, the test results will be normal. An alternative is monitoring basal body temperature—a method many believe is more sensitive and illuminating. The basal body temperature test is a naturopathic medical approach to accurately identifying thyroid problems. And best of all, it is easy to do at home—all you need is a thermometer.

Step one: Place a glass or instant-read digital thermometer beside your bed before you go to sleep.

Step two: As soon as you wake up in the morning, before you even get out of bed, place the glass thermometer under your armpit for a full 10 minutes, or place the digital thermometer under your tongue until it beeps, indicating that it has reached temperature. Move as little as possible while you wait, just lie there and rest with your eyes closed.

Step three: Read the thermometer and record the temperature, date, and time.

Step four: Repeat this process at least three mornings in a row, ideally at the same time.

Note: Menstruating women should perform the test on the second, third, and fourth days of menstruation.

A temperature between 97.6 and 98.2 is considered normal. Temperatures below that range could indicate hypothyroidism. Temperatures above 98.6 are less common but could indicate hyperthyroidism. For more information about the process, to interpret results, and for treatment options, see a naturally oriented healthcare professional.

The thyroid gland can also enlarge if it becomes too active, producing excessive amounts of hormones. Too much of these powerful hormones revs up metabolism, causing insomnia, nervousness, irritability, inability to gain weight, menstrual problems, and eventually chronic fatigue. This condition is known as hyperthyroidism.

Proper thyroid function and hormone activity levels are intricately connected. If the thyroid is not functioning properly, many important body functions are negatively influenced, including metabolism.

MIGHTY METABOLISM

If your body were a car, your thyroid gland would be what's pressing on the gas pedal. Metabolism is how fast the car moves. One of the most critical functions the thyroid performs is regulating metabolism. Metabolism is the building up, tearing down, and transformation of chemical energy into the mechanical energy that enables us to function. Metabolism affects bone health, liver function, menstruation, blood sugar control, and digestion, to name a few functions. It helps the body efficiently process and use the food we eat. Metabolism is often linked to weight loss or gain, but it also influences heart health, brain function, and immunity. That's why it is so critical to maintain healthy metabolism. When the thyroid gland is weak, sluggish, or not functioning properly, metabolism problems manifest. If prolonged stress goes unabated, altered metabolism function can have far-reaching health effects, including negatively affecting bone health and hormone balance.

In addition to the four thyroid hormones (T1, T2, T3, and T4), the thyroid gland produces calcitonin, a hormone that accelerates calcium absorption by bones. The parathyroid produces the appropriately named parathyroid hormone (PTH), which pulls calcium out. These hormones balance each other so there is an equal amount of bone deconstruction and reconstruction. If there is an imbalance, bone metabolism will be affected, and osteoporosis can occur.

Poor thyroid function and sluggish metabolism also can cause estrogen dominance, which often manifests as PMS, endometriosis, uterine fibroids, and infertility. The thyroid gland works with your adrenal glands and your ovaries to control your hormones. In addition to thyroid hormones, the gland also directs your body to produce progesterone. Insufficient thyroid function can result in reduced progesterone production, which contributes to PMS symptoms. Correcting estrogen dominance and supporting thyroid function results in restored metabolism, as well as symptom relief.

DAMAGING HEALTH EFFECTS OF STRESS

When stress is constant with no relief for days, weeks, or even months, the resulting hormonal imbalance increases the risk of serious diseases such as cancer and heart disease. Before that, we become symptomatic as we develop stress-related illnesses that can affect the

- gastrointestinal system (irritable bowel syndrome, colitis, ulcers, and indigestion),
- brain (headache/migraine, depression, clinical anxiety, and insomnia),
- immune system (frequent colds), and
- female reproductive system (uterine fibroids, absence of menstruation or abnormal bleeding, endometriosis, infertility, loss of libido, or heightened menopausal symptoms).

THYROID SUPPORT

The two best strategies for supporting your thyroid are healthy dietary choices and savvy supplementation. Diet truly is the foundation for health. What you eat affects your metabolism. Simple carbohydrates in the form of sugary foods, white flour, and junk foods are metabolized quickly. The resultant surge in glucose causes more insulin than necessary to be released into the bloodstream. Excess insulin is stored as fat; excess fat contributes to weight gain and estrogen dominance. Conversely, complex carbohydrates, such as whole grains, nuts, seeds, fruits, and legumes, are metabolized more slowly; glucose enters the bloodstream gradually and doesn't cause such an intense insulin reaction. You benefit from a steady supply of energy, and your bodily systems benefit because they aren't being exposed to extremes.

In addition to healthful dietary choices, you can support your thyroid with specific nutrients. Your comprehensive multivitamin should contain zinc; vitamins A, C, E; and the B vitamins. They are beneficial for thyroid health, and you rarely need more than what is provided in a good multivitamin. Other nutrients, including vitamin D, iodine, L-tyrosine, and selenium, either aren't present in a multivitamin or are required in doses greater than what is typically present in a vitamin. There have been several clinical studies indicating they can contribute to peak thyroid function.

Vitamin D has been shown to help balance PTH, which is significantly involved with bone health. Results of a study involving elderly women and another featuring adolescent females both indicated vitamin D helped balance PTH levels and enhanced bone health. In another study published in the *American Journal of Clinical Nutrition*, researchers associated obesity with decreased vitamin D bioavailability, which led to excessive PTH secretion.

Iodine is integral to thyroid function. Without it the gland cannot manufacture its hormones. Results of a study published in the *European Journal of Clinical Nutrition* showed that loss of iodine via breast milk among nursing women living in a mildly iodine-deficient area inhibited thyroid function. Iodine uses the amino acid L-tyrosine to convert T4 to the more powerful and active T3. Some studies also indicate that mercury (commonly found in dental fillings) negatively affects thyroid function because it displaces selenium, resulting in low levels of T3.

L-tyrosine is an amino acid found in meat proteins, almonds, avocados, bananas, dairy products, lima beans, pumpkin seeds, and sesame seeds. It is used to make several neurotransmitters, which are chemicals that help the nervous system and brain function. L-tyrosine is a precursor to norepinephrine and dopamine, which regulate mood. It also attaches to iodine to form active thyroid hormones. L-tyrosine levels are occasionally low in depressed people and those with kidney diseases. Supplementation is rarely necessary, but make sure your diet contains sufficient tyrosine-rich foods to help support thyroid function.

Selenium is a trace mineral. The body uses it to create an enzyme called glutathione peroxidase, which is an antioxidant. Glutathione works with vitamin E to protect cells from from free radical damage. Selenium plays a role in thyroid hormone metabolism as well. Severe selenium deficiency is a possible cause of goiter. However, supplementing with selenium if you aren't deficient can further impair thyroid function. There is no evidence that supplementing with selenium helps people with hypothyroidism who are not selenium deficient. Brazil nuts are the best source of selenium. Yeast, whole grains, and seafood are also good sources. Make sure your diet includes some of these selenium-rich foods.

Diet and supplementation are only part of the equation. If you are leading a stressful life that is causing your adrenal and thyroid glands to malfunction, causing various immediate symptoms and long-term health concerns, you cannot overlook the stress in your life. Adjusting your diet may help, but chances are if you are stressed out, you will not be able to stay committed to healthful eating. To keep your body in balance and your health intact, you must take measures to reduce the stress in your life or find healthy ways to cope with it.

SYMPTOMS OF STRESS

The Harvard Medical School Family Health Guide (Simon & Schuster, 1999) has identified these symptoms of stress separated by body function.

Physical
- Headache
- Back pain, tight neck and shoulders
- Indigestion and/or stomach pain
- Racing heart

Behavioral
- Increase in smoking or alcohol consumption
- Grinding teeth
- Bossiness
- Compulsive eating
- Inability to get things done

Emotional
- Crying
- Nervousness and/or edginess
- Loneliness
- Sense of powerlessness

Cognitive
- Trouble thinking clearly
- Forgetfulness
- Inability to make decisions
- Thoughts of escape
- Lack of creativity
- Incessant worrying

Listen to your body. If you recognize yourself in this list, make the effort to reduce stress.

STRESS RELIEF

The bedrock of any stress-relief plan is rest. Physiologically speaking, rest helps our bodies cope, rebound, and repair during times of heightened stress. In addition to finding time each day to rest, there are other stress-relieving techniques to try. Use what works for you. No matter what helps you relax, the most critical step is to make the effort.

I know from personal experience the importance of incorporating relaxation time into a hectic schedule. For example, I love music. As a past musician, I was exposed to music all the time. Music soothes me, so the stress from my busy practice necessitates I make time for music. It is the same with yoga. Although my intense travel schedule pulls me away from my regular yoga class, the practice is a necessary part of my stress-relief plan.

Music and yoga work for me, but they may not be right for you. Create a stress-relief plan that fits your personal interests. Here are some helpful hints that have worked for my patients.

Exercise. Walking, stretching, working out at the gym, and other physical activities help ease stress by releasing feel-good hormones called endorphins. Some of my patients use exercise time to clear thoughts, not think about problems, and focus solely on the activity, while others use it as a time to process problems. Either way, physical activity is a great stress reliever.

Fun. Find ways to have fun. Rent a funny movie, relax with friends, or enjoy the great outdoors. Add this item to your weekly "to do" list: Have some fun!

Emotional support. Psychotherapy and counseling can provide professional support; journaling, guided imagery, and self-talk are things you can do on your own. It is important to express yourself. Bottled-up anger, anxiety, fear, and other emotions can have a physical effect; they increase blood pressure, cause headaches, and can lead to ulcers. Get the help you need to confront conflict in an open and constructive manner.

Aromatherapy. All of our senses are involved in healing, and aromatherapy taps the sense of smell. Putting lavender drops on your pillow at night or burning incense or calming candles may be a great end-of-day ritual for you.

Meditation. Some of my patients report meditation helps them relax tense muscles, stop their minds from racing, and feel calm. There is scientific documentation to substantiate their reactions. The *American Journal of Health Promotion* reported "mindfulness meditation" significantly decreased the effects of daily hassles, psychological distress, and medical symptoms associated with stress. Look for tapes or local classes and be patient—meditation takes practice.

Diet. The best way to support your health is to follow healthy diet and lifestyle guidelines. If, as you read these words, you tune out thinking, "I have to change my diet, but healthy food is so boring," try again. Make a pampering ritual out of evening meals when you can. Serve your organic, whole-foods meal on the good dishes and set candles on the table. Savor the flavors and think about their nourishing and healing qualities. Your commitment to a healthy diet is too important to brush aside—it is your foundation.

Just say no. Sometimes it pays to be selfish with your time and energy. We have been programmed to think selfishness is a negative trait. If you don't take time for yourself, you may not be healthy enough to take time for others. Learn to say "no" every now and then.

REST AND REPAIR

Our bodies go through a variety of complex reactions when we are faced with stress. Stress is normal, and we are designed to adapt. When we rest, for example, our bodies can repair and rebound. But unrelenting stress with no downtime causes problems. Constant stress, when combined with a poor diet, negative lifestyle habits, and unhealthy digestion, can result in hormonal imbalance and cause serious health issues. Supporting the adrenals and thyroid—key glands of the endocrine system—is so important. If our bodies are unable to adapt internally, we become symptomatic. These symptoms become even more pronounced during times of hormonal change. The end result can be varied and dramatic.

CHAPTER 6

The End Result

C hange is inevitable—not only in life, but also in health. Change truly is the only thing that stays the same. We cannot stop change, but we can influence its effect on us. Women experience natural hormonal shifts throughout their lives. The only thing certain about hormonal activity is that it will change.

The point I hope I've made thus far is that proper endocrine and digestive function, which are intimately connected to each other and also related to diet and lifestyle, are paramount to health and hormone balance. If these systems aren't functioning optimally, you are likely to experience symptoms of hormone imbalance—most commonly estrogen dominance. Estrogen dominance is causing a broad range of women's health issues, including an increasing incidence of PMS, endometriosis, uterine fibroids, ovarian cysts, infertility, and menopausal symptoms. During times of hormonal change, these symptoms can intensify. These symptoms and illnesses are not normal or inevitable. They are *not* part of the aging process. They are the end result of various combined factors, including increased exposure to xenoestrogens, unhealthy diet and lifestyle activities, poor digestion, and excessive stress.

Regardless of what your symptoms have been labeled, they likely are caused by a state of estrogen dominance. What follows is a look at the possible end results of the various ways estrogen dominance can manifest.

PREMENSTRUAL SYNDROME

Although menstrual problems have become commonplace, it is not normal to have a painful period, irregular bleeding, or increased anxiety or depression before menstruation. The normal menstrual cycle is intricately balanced to ensure consistent hormonal activity. When there is hormonal imbalance, menstrual difficulties, most commonly PMS, can result.

Approximately 75 percent of menstruating women have some form of PMS. It is classified as PMS if symptoms occur anywhere from two to 14 days before menstruation. The timing of the symptoms is more important in identifying PMS than the symptoms themselves. PMS symptoms can vary in intensity and number with each menstrual cycle. They occur nearly every month and are absent during bleeding.

PMS SYMPTOMS

A wide range of symptoms is associated with PMS. Here are the most common.
- Anxiety
- Back pain
- Bloating
- Breast tenderness
- Change in libido
- Confusion
- Cramping
- Cravings for sweets
- Depression
- Headache
- Increased appetite
- Insomnia
- Irritability
- Mood swings
- Nervous tension
- Weight gain

About 3 percent of women with PMS have symptoms so severe they interrupt quality of life. In conventional medicine, severe PMS has been categorized as a disease called premenstrual dysphoric disorder (PMDD). I understand some women can experience this severe form of PMS, but it is ridiculous to label these women with a mental disorder and then prescribe antidepressants.

Regardless of severity, PMS is caused by a hormone imbalance. Initially, many believed progesterone to be the culprit, because its levels are highest just before menstruation. However, women with PMS typically have lower than normal progesterone levels during this time. Low progesterone levels when they are supposed to be high points to estrogen dominance. Because progesterone counters many of estrogen's potential side effects, it is easy to see what's triggering PMS.

Your healthcare provider can measure your serum or salivary progesterone levels. This is typically done between days 18 and 25 of your cycle. Inadequate progesterone—or too much estrogen—affects the endocrine system and results in the complex symptomatology of PMS.

PMS SOLUTIONS

Premenstrual syndrome is a multifaceted condition that may need more than one approach to reclaim monthly hormonal normalcy. Consider the following.

Nutrition
- Increase fiber consumption. Fiber binds to estrogen in the intestines so it can be efficiently eliminated.
- Eat less red meat. Cattle are often fed hormones, including estrogen, to fatten them for slaughter. These hormones are in the meat you eat and contribute to hormone imbalance.
- Reduce xenoestrogen exposure. Avoid processed foods, foods stored or heated in plastic, and other sources of man-made estrogens that may make their way into your meals. Support your body after discontinuing birth control pills as your system rebalances.

Lifestyle
- Reduce stress. Stress is known for causing menstrual irregularities.
- Exercise. Regular exercise is good for the body, mind, and spirit. Movement oxygenates the blood, keeps digestion moving smoothly, and improves mental outlook, to name a few benefits.

Complementary Medicine
- Consult a naturopathic physician, herbalist, acupuncturist, massage therapist, or light therapist. All of these healing methods can help women with PMS.

PERIMENOPAUSE

During the past several years, I have noticed a new diagnosis in the scientific literature: Perimenopause has become an overnight phenomenon. The reality is, however, that perimenopause is no more of an illness than menopause. These are both natural stages of physical development. Perimenopause is simply the nomenclature assigned to a set of symptoms and conditions that women of a specific age group—mid-30s to mid-40s—are having.

Experiencing some hormonal fluctuations as we age is normal. Menstruation, for example, becomes more erratic in some women before menopause. The ebb and flow of hormonal activity during this time can cause some symptoms as the body adapts. As the ovaries produce less estrogen, the adrenal glands are designed to pick up the pace and produce more if they are healthy. Although the estrogen produced in the adrenals is not as powerful as estrogen from the ovaries, it still has influence. These hormonal shifts are all a part of a natural process marking the end of our reproductive years. When our internal systems are working properly, this transition time is uneventful and a representation of normal physiology.

The increasing prevalence of estrogen dominance, however, has caused more women to experience a variety of uncomfortable and potentially dangerous symptoms associated with the years preceding menopause. Women are experiencing symptoms at younger ages than before. Menopausal symptoms can begin when a woman is in her 30s—nearly two decades before menopause.

As a result of the harmful ratio of estrogen to progesterone, women categorized as being perimenopausal can experience intense PMS symptoms (even if they have never had PMS before), irritability, anxiety, depression, anger, tearfulness, heart palpitations, and weight gain. In addition, many of the women who come to me previously diagnosed as perimenopausal also struggle with endometriosis, uterine fibroids, ovarian cysts, fibrocystic breasts, or infertility. All of these conditions are associated with increased tissue growth, a hallmark of estrogen dominance.

Endometriosis is one of the most common gynecological diseases affecting women today. The Endometriosis Research Center reports that more than 70 million women and girls worldwide have this condition. Medically, endometriosis symptoms occur when parts of the endometrium are scattered in the fallopian tubes, the outer surface of the uterus, on other pelvic organs, and various places they don't belong. With every monthly cycle, all these endometrial pieces respond to the hormonal signals from the ovaries. That is, they increase in size, fill with blood, and bleed at menstruation. This bleeding causes inflammation and pain.

Pain is the hallmark symptom of endometriosis. Often misdiagnosed as painful periods, endometriosis can cause pain in the low back, pelvis, and intestines and discomfort during or after intercourse. The severe pain can sometimes radiate down the legs and may be present during urination or bowel movements. About 30 percent to 40 percent of women with endometriosis have difficulty getting pregnant. Women who do not experience the severe pain associated with endometriosis may not be diagnosed until they seek treatment for infertility.

Endometriosis is difficult to diagnose, and its cause is unclear. There are several theories about its cause, including retrograde menstruation, immune system malfunctions, xenoestrogens, stress, and estrogen excess. A hormone balancing diet and lifestyle can often ease some of the discomfort if not eliminate it.

Uterine fibroids are the most common noncancerous tumors found in women of childbearing age. These fibrous masses can vary in size. About one-third of women with fibroids have abnormal bleeding, which can include heavy bleeding or bleeding between periods. Uterine fibroids are also associated with pain, a feeling of fullness, infertility, or multiple miscarriages. In the United States, uterine fibroids are the most common reason for hysterectomy. This surgical procedure should be avoided, especially because fibroids are considered another manifestation of estrogen dominance. Bringing hormones back into balance can often obviate even the need to surgically remove the fibroid. From a naturopathic perspective, fibroids are caused by estrogen excess from bowel toxicity, liver congestion, and xenoestrogen exposure. Subclinical hypothyroidism may be another contributing cause.

Polycystic ovaries occur when the ovaries enlarge and cysts form. The cysts are sacs that can contain fluid, semifluid, or solid matter. Worldwide statistics indicate that more than 20 percent of women of reproductive age have polycystic ovaries. Symptoms can include painful menstruation, abnormal menstruation, excessive body hair, obesity, and infertility. Results of a recent study featured in the American Heart Association's journal *Circulation* demonstrated that women with polycystic ovaries had a significantly higher risk of developing heart disease and stroke.

Polycystic ovary is another condition of hormone imbalance. When cysts are present, FSH and LH production can be altered, causing incomplete follicular development without consistent ovulation. Because the hormone system operates as a feedback loop, if one hormone is at an abnormal level, all related hormones are affected. Specifically, LH levels can be higher than normal, resulting in an increased LH to FSH ratio. The elevated LH levels result in a shift in ovarian hormone production toward increased estrogen levels. Estrogen stimulates cyst growth, and reduced estrogen causes them to shrink. Bringing the estrogen to progesterone ratio back into balance typically shrinks cysts.

Fibrocystic breasts are diagnosed in about 60 percent of women in their reproductive years, according to the American Cancer Society. This is a noncancerous condition characterized by one or more lumps in one or both breasts. The breast tissue feels thick, lumpy, or as if there are tiny beads scattered throughout the breasts. In addition to the lumpiness, breasts can be swollen, painful, and tender. Typically, symptoms are worse just before menstruation. The degree of discomfort can vary and usually subsides near the end of menstruation. By bringing estrogen and progesterone back into balance, fibrocystic breasts can often be cleared.

Infertility, technically diagnosed if there is an inability to conceive a child within one year, can also be attributed to estrogen dominance. One theory is that too much estrogen stimulates the ovaries to overproduce follicles. Over time this, combined with delayed childbearing, often results in infertility caused by follicle burnout, which is characterized by anovulatory cycles. During an anovulatory cycle, no egg is released and so no progesterone is produced, further contributing to estrogen imbalance. In addition, other estrogen-dominance disorders can cause infertility, including endometriosis, ovarian cysts, and thyroid dysfunction.

Estrogen dominance causes hormonal imbalance that can lead to menstrual difficulties, endometriosis, uterine fibroids, polycystic ovaries, fibrocystic breasts, and infertility. Birth control pills are often prescribed for severe cases of PMS, fibroids, and endometriosis, but taking prescription estrogen compounds the problem. The birth control pill is a combination of estrogen and progestin designed to prevent ovulation. Lack of ovulation prevents pregnancy, but ovulation ensures progesterone levels rise, keeping estrogen in check. Similar to using HRT for menopausal symptoms, using the birth control pill for these perimenopausal conditions compounds the problem of estrogen dominance. Just as hormone imbalance can cause problems during perimenopause, the symptoms of menopause can be magnified if a woman enters the change with a hormone imbalance. A woman's hormones are going to change at menopause, but if they are out of balance to begin with and combined with exhausted adrenals, her transition will be less than smooth.

MENOPAUSE

Menopause refers to the permanent cessation of menstrual cycles. Cycles stop when ovarian function gradually decreases, a result of diminished estrogen and progesterone levels. Menopause, I cannot stress enough, is *not* a disease; it is a normal, natural process. The female body is innately capable of achieving or maintaining optimal health and vitality throughout various changes during a lifetime. Supporting the body before, during, and after menopause can result in a nearly seamless transition.

Menopause can occur between the ages of 35 and 58, but the average age is 51. With female life expectancy at about 81 years, most women can expect to live one-third of their lives after menopause. Every day 5,400 North American women enter menopause. It is estimated that in less than 20 years, nearly 50 percent of the adult female population in the United States will be menopausal. With such significant numbers, it's not surprising menopause has become a key national health issue, or that pharmaceutical companies are so interested in developing drugs to "treat" it.

Between the huge numbers of potential customers and the increasing number of women reporting more severe symptoms associated with their menopausal transition, it is no wonder that menopause symptom relief has become such a big business for pharmaceutical and natural products companies alike. But why are so many women having trouble with this natural transition? Not all women have menopausal symptoms, and the menopausal complaints of women in industrialized countries are nearly unheard of in third-world countries. The symptoms I commonly see in my clinical practice include hot flashes, irritability, insomnia, rheumatism, and decreased energy. Other common symptoms include vaginal dryness, decreased libido, water retention, weight gain, headaches, fatigue, thinning of scalp hair, sleep disturbances, lack of concentration or memory lapses, and general body aches. I believe the evidence for these increased symptoms points to estrogen dominance, not estrogen deficiency as purveyors of HRT would have women believe.

At menopause, estrogen levels do decrease, but only between 40 percent and 50 percent. Progesterone levels, however, can drop to nearly zero, according to John R. Lee, MD, in *What Your Doctor May Not Tell You About Menopause* (Warner Books, 1996). As I've explained, the interrelationship between hormones is a delicate one. When one of these hormones becomes too prevalent, the body becomes more sensitive to the opposing one. When estrogen levels are high, the body is sensitized to progesterone. When progesterone levels drop at menopause, estrogen dominates, causing the list of uncomfortable symptoms many menopausal women experience.

Despite this, during the past several decades, conventional medical doctors have come to view HRT as the obvious choice for menopausal women. These artificial hormones often reduce some symptoms, but not all. Recently, substantial scientific evidence has confirmed that side effects of HRT far outweigh the benefits. Unopposed estrogen can exacerbate some menopausal symptoms, including mood swings and body aches, because estrogen alters cellular function. It has serious health implications as well, including increasing endometrial and breast cancer risk.

THE HRT MYTH

For more than five decades, the estrogen replacement drug Premarin, made from the urine of pregnant mares, was billed as the menopausal cure-all. Advertisements claimed it would keep women forever young. Even though many clinical studies published in peer-reviewed medical journals questioned the safety of Premarin and other similar drugs, physicians throughout the United States continued to push it. Why? It is a quick fix and it has become big business.

According to a report in *JAMA*, 46 million prescriptions were written for Premarin in 2000 alone, making it the second most frequently prescribed drug in the United States. That added up to more than $1 billion in sales for one drug. The newer drug, Prempro, combines estrogen and progestin (synthetic progesterone); more than 22 million prescriptions were written for it in 2000.

WOMEN'S HEALTH INITIATIVE (WHI) STUDY RESULTS

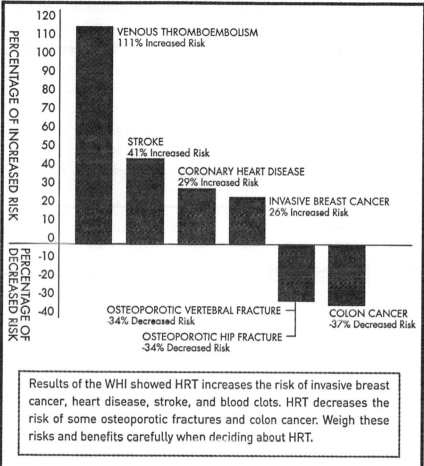

Results of the WHI showed HRT increases the risk of invasive breast cancer, heart disease, stroke, and blood clots. HRT decreases the risk of some osteoporotic fractures and colon cancer. Weigh these risks and benefits carefully when deciding about HRT.

Recently, the Women's Health Initiative (WHI) study demonstrated that Prempro does the opposite of what the drug companies claimed it would do. Results showed HRT increases the risk of invasive breast cancer, heart disease, stroke, and blood clots. Because of these dangers, the study was discontinued early. Follow-up evaluations of the WHI indicate HRT also increases ovarian cancer risk.

Previously, women were led to believe HRT would not only alleviate their menopausal symptoms, but the drugs would also protect them from heart disease and strengthen their bones. In fact, some women who were not even experiencing menopausal symptoms went on the drug for those reasons. But estrogen therapy doesn't appear to help protect against osteoporosis, either. Results of a study published in the *New England Journal of Medicine* revealed estrogen use by women older than 65 had no benefit in preventing hip fracture. Other research shows estrogen may decrease bone breakdown, but it doesn't increase bone production; in fact, it eventually causes bone production to decrease. With regard to HRT and heart disease, there have been no controlled clinical studies proving hormone therapy improves cardiovascular health. Studies featured in *JAMA* indicate HRT also causes abnormal menstrual bleeding and changes in breast tissue. HRT also causes increased breast density, which can decrease mammography sensitivity and effectiveness.

QUITTING HRT

So you're looking at your Premarin (or other HRT) prescription with much more suspicion now. The health risks for you are enough reason to doubt, and that's not even broaching the less-than-humane production processes used to create the drug. You're probably wondering how to get off HRT safely. First, you should consult your healthcare provider. I don't advise discontinuing a prescription medication without first informing your prescribing physician. I fully promote patient empowerment, but find a supportive provider who will supervise your transition from HRT to either natural alternatives or off therapy all together. With diet and lifestyle modifications, often combined with natural remedies, you can be free from HRT.

Women clearly have been misled and misinformed about HRT. As a result, although this treatment has alleviated some of women's day-to-day discomforts, it has put them at increased risk of heart disease and cancer. This is a clear indication of how the medical community has at times abandoned the sacred oath "first do no harm." We should never trade symptom relief for significant long-term risk. Wise women will avoid HRT and use it only as a treatment of last resort. In some rare cases, a prescription drug may be necessary for a short time. Based on the scientific research, however, HRT should never be used long-term under any circumstance.

ANOTHER TREATMENT OF LAST RESORT

Too many women are taking HRT unnecessarily and are having adverse health effects. In addition to this medical travesty, too many women are being told they need hysterectomies to treat their various complaints. Half a million women have this surgery each year. One in three women will have a hysterectomy by the time she is 60. Women in the United States are four times more likely to have a hysterectomy than women in Europe, New Zealand, and Australia are. These surgeries are big business with costs exceeding $5 billion each year.

The surgery is sometimes prescribed to prevent uterine or ovarian cancer. The theory is if the organ is prone to disease and it isn't being used, remove it and the potential for cancer. However, ovarian cancer is rare— only 4 percent of women will get it. It seems a ludicrous practice to remove what might become cancerous.

Another common reason for a hysterectomy is fibroids. Michael Glassner, MD, medical director for reproductive medicine at Bryn Mawr Hospital in Pennsylvania, says fibroid cases rarely require hysterectomy. Of the 600,000 women counseled by the Hysterectomy Educational Resources and Services organization who were told they needed a hysterectomy, 98 percent did not need the surgery.

As you can see, many hysterectomies are unnecessary. Results of a study featured in *Obstetrics and Gynecology* showed 75 percent of the hysterectomies evaluated were "recommended inappropriately." The effects are beyond monetary for the women involved. The surgery can cause lifelong side effects. Sexual desire and pleasure are severely diminished after hysterectomy, if not lost completely. Immunity also suffers from the absence of the uterus. It produces prostaglandins, which are hormonelike substances that regulate various physiological responses, including inflammation, muscle contraction, vascular dilation, and platelet aggregation. Cardiovascular disease risk can increase because of this lost protection. The *American Journal of Cardiology* reported that women with hysterectomies had a higher risk of heart attack or coronary death. Also, when the uterus is removed, ovarian function is reduced, which alters hormone production. Hysterectomy also increases risk of depression and osteoporosis.

A hysterectomy should only be performed if cancer has been diagnosed or in life-threatening situations. It is not indicated for prolapsed uterus, sterilization, or excessive menstrual bleeding—the top three reasons for the surgery, according to the Mayo Clinic. My advice to women who have been told they need a hysterectomy is to get a second opinion.

CYCLES OF LIFE

We are designed to easily move from one life cycle to the next. From puberty through menopause, we come full circle, closing the feminine loop to live one-third of our lives in wisdom and power. This process does not need to be medically managed or surgically expedited. Outside influences can and often do affect our ability to make smooth transitions. Whether those influences are a persuasive doctor waving an HRT prescription and making lavish promises, or simply diet and lifestyle factors affecting well-being, the end result is an increasing number of symptoms and conditions associated with an imbalance of estrogen and progesterone that affect all hormonal activity. Although symptom relief is important, addressing the underlying cause is necessary. Natural solutions can help accomplish both.

CHAPTER 7

Natural Relief

So we find ourselves at a transition point in our lives—perhaps in our late 30s, or maybe facing menopause in our 50s—and we are experiencing discomforts. In my case, it was a menstrual cycle I didn't recognize as my own, complete with mood swings and cramping. If we approach conventional medicine for answers or relief, we will likely be handed a prescription for synthetic hormones. Our challenge, in the face of prevailing medical practice and profit-driven pharmaceutical companies, is to find healthcare that honors a woman's bodily wisdom and her cycles of life, healthcare that respects female physiology and is not intent on medicalizing and pathologizing natural hormone cycles. You'll be going against the grain in your quest, but there are practitioners who can offer natural, gentle approaches for addressing hormone imbalance—the root of symptoms such as PMS, hot flashes, and lost libido. These remedies provide symptom relief while also helping treat the underlying cause and prevent serious health risks. Unlike HRT, they work with your body, not against it.

In light of the results of the Women's Health Initiative, which showed HRT drugs increase cancer and heart disease risk, there is a dramatic, renewed interest in natural alternatives that address women's health issues. Scientific research on natural substances is increasing, as is consumer demand. More information and more choices are available to you now than before. If you are committed to working to rebalance your hormones and, in the meantime, find natural symptom relief, the remedies that follow for hot flashes and night sweats; mood, energy, and well-being; sleep and relaxation; lost libido; and breast fibroids are definitely worth knowing about.

HOT FLASHES AND NIGHT SWEATS

One of the most common symptoms associated with menopause is an erratic internal thermostat. As many as 75 percent to 85 percent of women approaching menopause experience hot flashes. These heat waves occur when peripheral blood vessels dilate, causing flushing and increased skin temperature. Although not life-threatening, hot flashes and night sweats are uncomfortable and irritating and can disrupt quality of life. Hot flashes are more prevalent in the first few years after menopause; as the body adapts to its new hormonal profile, they typically dissipate.

The most widely used and thoroughly studied herbal extract for menopause is **black cohosh** (*Cimicifuga racemosa*). This herb is an approved treatment in Europe for premenstrual discomfort, painful periods, and numerous menopausal symptoms, including hot flashes and night sweats. In a double-blind study, 80 patients took black cohosh, conjugated estrogens, or placebo for 12 weeks. Black cohosh produced greater improvement in vaginal lining and

> **Black cohosh**
> (*Cimicifuga racemosa*)
> • 40 mg/day
> • hot flashes/night sweats, vaginal dryness, PMS, hormone rebalancing

better results on a scale for menopausal complaints and an index for rating anxiety than did estrogens or placebo. The daily number of hot flashes experienced among the women taking black cohosh dropped from an average of five to just one. Other studies have shown black cohosh to improve ringing in the ears, heart palpitations, profuse perspiration, vertigo, nervousness, irritability, and headache.

Black cohosh can bind to receptor sites without changing hormone levels, but it is not a phytoestrogen. Researchers conducting cell studies have found that black cohosh appears to protect against breast tumor cell growth; it doesn't stimulate tumor growth. So black cohosh is considered safe and effective even for women who are at high risk of developing estrogen-dependent cancers. The dose of black cohosh is 40 mg per day, standardized to contain 2.5 percent triterpene glycosides calculated as 27-deoxyactein. This is the compound and dose used in the many clinical studies. Black cohosh is safe for long-term use based on results of current research.

In addition to black cohosh, isoflavones from **soy** can help cool hot flashes and reduce high cholesterol, bone loss, and breast cancer risk. Isoflavones are phytoestrogens, or plant estrogens. Their effects in the body are similar to estrogen, but weaker. They can latch onto the same receptor sites and prevent stronger, more harmful estrogens from doing so. This way, when there is too much estrogen in the body, they help block its influence. When there isn't enough, isoflavones can help by offering a modest estrogenic effect.

> **Soy**
> • 40 g/day or more
> • hot flashes/night sweats, vaginal dryness, PMS, hormone rebalancing

Soy protein from food sources can help reduce hot flashes and other menopausal symptoms. In a double-blind, placebo-controlled study, researchers working with 104 women found soy protein provided significant relief from hot flashes compared with placebo. The women who ate what amounted to 60 grams of soy protein a day had 26 percent fewer hot flashes after three weeks and 45 percent fewer hot flashes after 12 weeks.

Be sure to distinguish between dietary soy isoflavones and synthetic supplement forms—they don't appear to have the same results. The best way to get soy's benefits is to eat more soy foods, including soy milk, miso, tempeh, fresh soy beans (edamame), tofu, and any of the myriad soy-based products available today. You also can replace cow's milk with soy milk in recipes or add powdered soy protein or silken tofu to smoothies to increase your intake. The typical amount of soy protein found in 2.5 cups of soy milk or one-half pound of tofu is 25 grams. Studies have used doses up to 40 grams daily.

Additional **vitamin E** may also be helpful in relieving hot flashes and night sweats. Results of several clinical studies from the 1940s show vitamin E effectively reduces hot flashes and vaginal discomforts. Check the

> **Vitamin E**
> • 800 IU/day
> • hot flashes/night sweats, vaginal dryness, PMS

amount provided by your multivitamin; I recommend 800 IU daily for women experiencing menopausal symptoms.

MOOD, ENERGY, WELL-BEING

In addition to poor energy levels, some menopausal women experience mood swings, irritability, depression, and anxiety. These women say they just don't feel right. Their overall well-being is negatively affected by their increased menopausal symptoms caused by hormone imbalance. Women do not have to suffer with these symptoms; there are several useful remedies for improving energy levels, mood, and well-being.

Ginseng (*Panax* spp) can help support the adrenal glands during times of stress, an important factor in rebalancing hormones. Some studies indicate ginseng can help reduce menopausal symptoms and improve mood and well-being. Although not all the science on ginseng is entirely convincing, small studies have shown the herb to improve energy and mental ability. I recommend *Panax ginseng* at a daily dose of 50 mg.

> **Ginseng** (*Panax* spp)
> • 50 mg/day
> • menopausal symptoms, mood, well-being, energy, hormone rebalancing

Green tea (*Camellia sinensis*) is one of my favorite herbs for women's health. It contains a small amount of caffeine, which supports stamina and reduces fatigue. Newer research also indicates green tea can stimulate metabolism to help avoid weight gain or contribute to weight loss. And in addition to green tea's having been shown in clinical studies to help prevent breast cancer, its overall antioxidant activity is important for generalized immune function. The recommended daily dose of green tea is 250 mg.

> **Green tea**
> (*Camellia sinensis*)
> • 250 mg/day
> • fatigue, metabolism, immunity

St. John's wort (*Hypericum perforatum*) is an effective herb for mild to moderate depression and anxiety associated with depression. It is a prescription antidepressant in Germany and a popular herbal remedy in the United States. In several randomized, double-blind, placebo-controlled studies, researchers concluded St. John's wort significantly benefits patients with mild to moderate depression without side effects. St. John's wort also has been found to be as effective as tricyclic antidepressant drugs (amitriptyline, imipramine, maprotiline), but the herb is more tolerable. In a review of 17 studies on St. John's wort and nine studies on fluoxetine (Prozac), researchers showed the herb was as effective as fluoxetine for treating mild depression.

> **St. John's wort**
> (*Hypericum perforatum*)
> • 300 mg three times/day
> • mild to moderate depression, fatigue, menopausal symptoms

This herb is not indicated for severe depression. In two fairly recent trials, researchers evaluated St. John's wort's efficacy against major and severe depression. Neither trial showed the herb to be an effective option for these types of depression.

Other research indicates St. John's wort is effective for fatigue and menopausal symptoms, however. Since it isn't known to cause side effects, it is safe to use for fatigue and mood. The standard dose is 300 mg three times a day. Find an extract standardized to 0.3 percent hypericin. If you are depressed, use this herb under the supervision of a healthcare provider. Depression can be dangerous; I don't advise switching from a prescription antidepressant to St. John's wort without the help of a knowledgeable practitioner.

A FRIENDLY REMINDER ABOUT NATURAL REMEDIES

The natural symptom-relieving herbs and nutrients featured in this chapter are not cure-alls or magic bullets. They work best when used in combination with a healthy diet and positive lifestyle modifications. Comprehensive support of the endocrine and digestive systems is also necessary.

We are all different with individual health needs. What works for one person may not work for another. I am reminded of this all of the time in my clinical practice. For example, I will see two women with the same previous diagnosis of perimenopause and completely different symptoms. The health plans I recommend are unique to each woman. To get specialized recommendations (and to avoid potentially harmful interactions), work with a qualified healthcare provider.

SLEEP AND RELAXATION

Insomnia is a common problem for women before, during, and even after menopause. Often, night sweats and hot flashes contribute to this problem by disrupting sleep patterns. Insomnia is defined by taking more than 30 minutes to get to sleep, waking up frequently throughout the night and having trouble getting back to sleep, or feeling groggy and tired when you wake. The National Center on Sleep Disorder Research reports 30 percent of patients seen by primary care physicians experience difficulties sleeping. Getting a deep, relaxing sleep each night is important to hormonal balance and overall health.

Over-the-counter and prescription sleep medications can cause side effects and contribute to morning grogginess. There are numerous effective natural alternatives. A few of my favorites include valerian, hops, kava, and L-theanine. They are most effective when taken about an hour before bedtime.

Results of clinical studies have shown **valerian** root extract (*Valeriana officinalis*) can help relieve insomnia, stress, and anxiety. In a placebo-controlled study, participants taking 600 mg valerian two hours before bedtime slept better than those taking placebo. In another study, researchers found that participants taking valerian before stressful situations reported less anxiety. The daily dose of valerian is 200 mg of the standardized extract containing 0.8 percent valerenic acid, the active compound. Valerian helps calm the nervous system, and I recommend it be combined with 100 mg of hops each evening. **Hops** (*Humulus lupulus*) can also help ease insomnia and anxiety. Because its sedative effect is quite mild, it is often combined with other herbs. The standard dose of hops is 0.5 grams taken up to three times a day for anxiety.

Kava (*Piper methysticum*) is commonly used to treat anxiety, but there is some evidence it can help with insomnia.

Researchers suggests kava relaxes the muscles in the body and increases alertness. In a six-week study, patients with stress-induced insomnia took 120 mg of kava daily. The herb reduced the time it took to fall asleep, increased the number of hours slept, and improved waking mood. In the same study, a combination of kava and valerian improved sleep slightly more effectively than either herb alone.

In another study, researchers compared kava to antianxiety benzo diazepine drugs in patients with generalized anxiety disorder. The 400 mg dose of kava was as effective as the pharmacuticals, but with fewer adverse effects.

Valerian
(*Valeriana officinalis*)
• 600 mg two hours before bedtime
• insomnia, anxiety

Hops
(*Humulus lupulus*)
• 100 mg taken with valerian before bedtime; or 0.5 g up to three times daily for anxiety
• insomnia, anxiety

Kava
(*Piper methysticum*)
• 210 mg one hour before bedtime for insomnia; 40–70 mg three times daily for anxiety (do not exceed 300 mg/day)
• insomnia, anxiety

Although kava is not addictive, it has come under scrutiny from the U.S. Food and Drug Administration after reports of kava-induced liver damage. These cases likely involved medication and/or alcohol use. Do not use kava in combination with medications that affect the liver or with alcohol or if you have an existing liver condition.

Kava is typically sold standardized to an amount of kavalactones per dose. For insomnia, take 210 mg of kavalactones one hour before bedtime. For anxiety, take 40 to 70 mg kavalactones three times daily; do not exceed 300 mg per day.

L-theanine is an amino acid found in green tea. It has been shown to increase brain waves that relate to alert relaxation. Not only does it promote relaxation, it also helps relieve stress. L-theanine reduces blood pressure and promotes muscle relaxation, helping the body calm down. L-theanine is ideal for women who have breakthrough insomnia, meaning they wake up during the night and cannot get back to sleep. Valerian and hops will help you fall asleep, and L-theanine will help you stay asleep without causing daytime drowsiness. The evening dosage of L-theanine is 50 mg.

L-Theanine
• 50 mg one hour before bedtime
• insomnia, relaxation, stress relief

Other natural insomnia remedies include **B vitamins** (be sure your multivitamin contains a comprehensive blend of B vitamins at doses greater than the recommended daily allowance [RDA]), a **calcium/magnesium** supplement taken at night, and **GABA** (gamma-aminobutyric acid). GABA is an amino acid produced in the brain that acts as a neurotransmitter (a chemical that fosters communication between nerve cells) and helps keep stress-related nerve impulses at bay. Various dietary and lifestyle factors can reduce the amount of GABA the brain produces, leading to anxiety, irritability, insomnia, and even depression. An hour or so before bedtime, take 500 to 1,000 mg. Its calming effect can help you fall asleep. If anxiety contributes to your sleep problems, take GABA along with valerian.

GABA
• 500–1,000 mg one hour before bedtime
• insomnia, anxiety

LOWERED LIBIDO

A common problem associated with hormonal imbalance is decreased desire to have sex. This can negatively affect self-esteem and overall well-being and decrease relationship intimacy. Many of the previously mentioned symptoms—hot flashes, decreased energy, and depression—can contribute to lost libido. Lowered levels of testosterone can cause lowered libido, because this androgenic hormone plays a significant role in sexual desire. Restoring adrenal function to help rebalance hormones can help increase testosterone levels in menopausal women.

Reducing stress and easing the other symptoms associated with hormonal imbalance also will help restore sexual desire. A woman's fluctuating hormones have far-reaching effects, including altered relationship dynamics. Psychological support or relationship counseling may be helpful during these times of change. Sexual arousal also has a strong emotional connection, particularly for women. As you go through change, you may need to communicate differently or more frequently with your partner regarding your sexual needs. As far as remedies go, many of my patients report *Panax ginseng* improves their interest in sex.

Ginkgo (*Ginkgo biloba*) may also help restore sexual desire in women. In one study involving women with antidepressant-induced sexual dysfunction, ginkgo was 84 percent effective. The herb enhanced desire,

> **Ginkgo**
> (*Ginkgo biloba*)
> • 209 mg/day
> • low libido

lubrication, orgasm, and resolution. The average dose in the open trial was 209 mg daily. In another study, researchers combined ginkgo with **Muira puama** and studied the effects of this combination on libido and sexual activity in premenopausal and postmenopausal women. The women taking the herbal supplement for

> **Muira puama**
> • 1.5 g/day
> • low libido

one month reported more frequent sexual desires, sexual intercourse, and sexual fantasies. They also reported improved satisfaction with sex life, ability to reach orgasm, intensity of orgasm, and intensity of sexual desire. These researchers are planning a double-blind trial to further explore the efficacy of this combination. The German Commission E rates *Muira puama* an unapproved herb with no documented risk and says it lacks scientific documentation for the uses claimed by the natural products industry. There are probably better remedies to try; consult an herbalist or naturopathic physician.

L-arginine, an amino acid, may also help improve libido. I recommend 5 to 6 grams daily to my patients. L-arginine was part of a combination product that showed promise when tested recently. Researchers gave the combo containing extracts of ginseng, ginkgo, and damiana (*Turnera aphrodisiaca*); L-arginine; multivitamins; and minerals to women older than 21 looking to improve their sexual function. After four weeks, 73.5 percent of the group taking the combination reported improved satisfaction with their overall sex lives compared with 37.2 percent of those taking placebo. The participants noted improvements in sexual desire, vaginal dryness, frequency of intercourse and orgasm, and clitoral stimulation.

> **L-Arginine**
> • 5–6 g/day
> • low libido

Although most of the research on **maca** (*Lepidium meyenii*) has been done in men with erectile dysfunction, there is reason to believe it can help women with low libido. I recommend a dose of 1,500 to 2,500 mg a day. I also advise my patients to take an **essential fatty acid** supplement—600 to 1,200 mg per day from fish oils—and to stay well hydrated.

> **Maca**
> (*Lepidium meyenii*)
> • 1,500–2,500 mg/day
> • low libido

> **Essential fatty acids**
> (from fish oils)
> • 600–1,200 mg/day
> • low libido

Vaginal dryness, irritation, and thinning often contribute to decreased sexual pleasure and, by extension, desire. Decreased estrogen levels typically contribute to these vaginal complaints. In addition to over-the-counter lubricants, several herbs can help restore the vaginal environment. In her *Women's Bodies, Women's Wisdom* (Bantam Books, 1998), Christiane Northrup, MD, recommends the botanicals **black cohosh, dandelion** (*Taraxacum officinale*), and **oats** (*Avena sativa*) for restoring vaginal lubrication. Take these herbs orally.

BREAST FIBROIDS

Fibrocystic breasts are associated with abnormal tissue growth caused by estrogen dominance. Women frequently find benign lumps in their breasts during their perimenopause years. To successfully alleviate this condition, work to normalize hormone balance. In the meantime, there are nutrients and herbs that can help.

SYMPTOM RELIEF SUMMARY

	Anxiety	Breast fibroids	Energy	Hot flashes/ night sweats	Insomnia	Low libido	Mood/ Well-being	PMS	Vaginal dryness
Black cohosh				X				X	X
B vitamins					X			X	
Calcium/ Magnesium					X			X	
Chaste tree		X						X	
Dandelion									X
EFAs						X			X
Evening primrose oil		X						X	
GABA	X				X				
Ginkgo						X			
Ginseng			X			X	X		
Green tea			X						
Hops	X				X				
Kava	X				X		X		
L-arginine						X			
L-theanine					X				
Maca						X			
Muira puama						X			
Oats									X
Soy				X					
St. John's wort							X		
Valerian	X				X				
Vitamin E		X		X				X	

Note: Consult a healthcare provider before taking any of the above-mentioned herbs or nutrients. Individualized recommendations and doses will be the best treatment for your body.

Vitamin E, at a dose of 400 to 600 IU daily, has been shown in several studies to reduce symptoms of fibrocystic breasts and PMS. Exactly how vitamin E works is unclear, but it helps normalize circulating hormones in women with fibrocystic breasts and PMS. It also normalizes elevated pituitary hormones (FSH and LH), which are common in women with fibrocystic breasts.

> **Vitamin E**
> • 400–600 IU/day
> • fibroids, PMS

The herb **chaste tree** (*Vitex agnus-castus*) is an effective herb for fibrocystic breasts, because it helps balance progesterone and estrogen levels by increasing progesterone production. Another theory is that chaste tree acts on the pituitary gland to suppress prolactin, a hormone that stimulates milk production in pregnant women. Elevated prolactin levels when milk production is not required can cause breast tenderness and other PMS symptoms. The recommended daily dose is 20 to 40 mg of chaste tree extract standardized to contain 0.5 percent agnuside, the active compound. Results may take a while, so be patient.

> **Chaste tree**
> (*Vitex agnus-castus*)
> • 20–40 mg/day
> • fibroids, breast tenderness, PMS

Evening primrose oil (*Oenothera biennis*) has been shown to alleviate symptoms of fibrocystic breasts as well as PMS and menopause. This herb is an accepted treatment for fibrocystic breasts in the United States and Europe. Daily supplementation was shown in a study published in the *Lancet* to produce substantial relief in 40 percent to 50 percent of women who take it. Results take several weeks or even months, so stick with it. The dose is typically 3 grams daily for cyclic breast pain. Take this supplement with food.

> **Evening primrose oil**
> (*Oenothera biennis*)
> • 3 g/day
> • fibroids, breast pain, PMS

Researchers also have shown a strong connection between caffeine consumption and fibrocystic breasts. Caffeine, theophylline, and theobromine are methylxanthines; they promote overproduction of cellular products, such as fibrous tissue and cyst fluid. Results of one study showed limiting sources of methylxanthines (coffee, tea, cola, chocolate, and caffeinated medications) dramatically improved fibrocystic breast conditions. Among women who abstained, 97.5 percent saw improvement. Among women who limited their consumption, 75 percent improved. Those who didn't change their diet to limit or eliminate methylxanthines showed little improvement.

DANGEROUS HEALTH RISKS

Symptom relief is important, but in addition to this, many of my patients are worried about fending off serious illnesses associated with times of hormonal change and aging. The goal of any comprehensive women's health program is not only to provide safe symptom relief and correct the underlying causes of said symptoms, but also to help prevent life-threatening diseases including cancer, osteoporosis, heart disease, and Alzheimer's disease.

CHAPTER 8

Preventing Other Illnesses

Addressing the underlying cause or causes of hormonal imbalance relieves symptoms while helping to prevent serious, life-threatening illnesses. Often, when we're feeling good, we take our health for granted. Getting a diagnosis or even just being told we are at risk for a serious illness, however, is not only frightening, it can cause us to take stock. When we face illness, we realize the true value of our health and its effect on the quality of our lives. The diseases women fear most as they age—beyond cancer, which I've already discussed in Chapter 3—are typically osteoporosis, Alzheimer's disease, and heart disease. All these illnesses have a strong connection to hormonal health. Tending to your hormones not only minimizes the discomforts I've already talked about, but it reduces your risk for more serious illnesses.

OSTEOPOROSIS

According to the National Osteoporosis Foundation, 10 million people presently have porous and fragile bones, and another 34 million have decreased bone mass, placing them at significant risk of developing osteoporosis. About 80 percent of those people are women. The organization reports 50 percent of women older than 50 will have an osteoporosis-related fracture in their lifetime. More than 3 million people are diagnosed with osteoporosis each year; half of them will suffer a fracture. It is time we understood our bones and started taking better care; the effort can equal extended quality of life in later years. Osteoporosis is not created overnight; it is the result of a lifetime of diet and lifestyle choices. Just as these factors contribute to hormone health and overall health, they also contribute to bone health.

Bone is living, dynamic tissue continually being reconstructed. To ensure bones stay healthy and strong, demolition and construction crews work around the clock. Osteoclasts are cells that break down old bone, and osteoblasts build new bone. When the activities of these two types of cells are balanced, bone mass is retained. Excessive osteoclast activity or decreased osteoblast activity results in bone loss and eventually osteoporosis.

DID YOU KNOW?

Bone is living tissue that remodels and regenerates 24 hours a day. In fact, every eight years, you have a whole new skeleton. By age 30, peak bone mass is determined. This makes it even more important to begin a bone-building program as early as possible.

Hormones, as I've mentioned, have a direct effect on bone health. The thyroid gland releases two hormones especially critical to the bone remodeling process. Parathyroid hormone (PTH) regulates blood calcium levels. When blood calcium levels are low, the thyroid releases more PTH. This hormone increases bone cell formation activity, which releases calcium into the blood and increases calcium absorption from the kidneys. As a result, more calcium is absorbed from the diet, and less is lost in urine.

The other hormone released by the thyroid gland is calcitonin. It balances the effects of PTH. If too much PTH is released because of low blood calcium levels, too much calcium is removed from the bones, which can make them weak. When blood calcium levels are too high, calcitonin reduces the rate at which calcium is released from the bones, increases the rate of calcium excreted by the kidneys, and reduces calcium absorption in the intestines.

If the thyroid is not functioning properly—if it is sluggish or weak—it will not be able to maintain an optimal balance of these two hormones. In addition, if you are not getting enough calcium in your diet, the body will take calcium from your bones. After all, osteoporosis is a survival mechanism. It is the body's way of defending against calcium deficiency. Not only is calcium important to bone health, it is vital to heart, nerve, and muscle function. Just as the adrenals will use progesterone to make cortisol to help us survive the onslaught of stress, our body will jeopardize bone health if it needs the calcium elsewhere.

Another hormone involved in bone health is estrogen, though to a much lesser degree than the aforementioned thyroid hormones. Estrogen stimulates calcitonin formation. Calcitonin increases calcium uptake by bones and inhibits bone breakdown. It is involved in the body's normal processes of bone maintenance. There is even much research to support estrogen therapy for stabilizing bone mass and perhaps increasing bone density in postmenopausal women. But faced with the choice of HRT for bone health, you would be wise to carefully evaluate your risk-to-benefit ratio. With the increased risk of heart disease and cancer from HRT, think carefully about using it to protect your bones. Estrogen therapy or HRT is not necessarily the solution to osteoporosis. In fact, your bones would be much better served by proper nutrition.

Several nutrients are necessary for proper bone formation and strength. Our bodies don't make these nutrients, so we must get them from diet, dietary supplements, or sunlight, as in the case of vitamin D. Vitamin D, calcium, magnesium, boron, vitamin K, and B vitamins are important to bone health, as are other trace minerals, including chromium, copper, zinc, and molybdenum.

A DANGEROUS COMBINATION

Results of a recent study from Denmark confirmed a connection between osteoporosis and heart disease. Researchers demonstrated that low bone-mineral density is a predictor of heart disease death among elderly women. They concluded severe osteoporosis in the hip might indicate advanced hardening of the arteries. This means women diagnosed with osteoporosis are at increased risk and need to be particularly diligent in protecting their hearts.

Calcium is an important component in preventing osteoporosis and slowing its progression. Women with osteoporosis are often deficient in both calcium and magnesium. Calcium is the key ingredient in bone building. Magnesium, on the other hand, plays an important role in maintaining bone mass.

Many studies confirm calcium enhances bone health. The question is typically what type of calcium to take and in what ratio with magnesium. For optimal absorption, I recommend a dietary supplement with a combination of calcium carbonate, calcium lactate, calcium citrate, and calcium chelate at a dose of at least 600 mg per day. This should be taken with about 250 mg of magnesium in the form of magnesium oxide and magnesium aspartate. Look for one tablet fitting this description to reduce the number of supplements you have to take. You can also enhance your intake by choosing calcium-rich foods, including dark green vegetables, nuts, seeds, fish canned with their bones (sardines, for example), and calcium-fortified orange juice and milk alternatives. I am not a big advocate of milk, cheese, and other dairy products because of their mucous-forming and hyperallergenic properties. You might want to limit your intake or avoid them altogether; there are plenty of other good sources of calcium. Magnesium can be found in kelp, wheat bran, wheat germ, almonds, cashews, blackstrap molasses, brewer's yeast, buckwheat, and whole grains. Other foods with less, but still significant amounts of, magnesium include collard and dandelion greens, dried fruit, avocados, and shrimp.

Vitamin D helps the body absorb calcium and keep PTH levels in check. Deficiency has been linked to excessive PTH secretion and to an increase in hip fractures and bone loss. Results of research indicate taking vitamin D with calcium results in better bone health than if either were taken alone. Vitamin D is safe at doses of 400 IU per day. Skin synthesizes vitamin D from sunlight, so try to get a little sun every day if possible. Food sources of vitamin D include cod liver oil, cold-water fish, butter, egg yolks, and fortified products.

Boron is a trace mineral that influences hormone metabolism. Results of animal studies indicate boron supplementation increases bone strength. Researchers also have suggested boron as a treatment for osteoporosis. Although they have yet to prove boron supplementation prevents or reverses bone loss, researchers have shown this mineral to decrease calcium loss. Good food sources of boron include raisins, prunes, noncitrus fruits, grains, leafy vegetables, and nuts. The typical diet provides adequate boron, so supplementation usually is unnecessary.

Vitamin K has a biochemical role in bone formation. Low blood levels of vitamin K are associated with osteoporosis. Several studies have shown this, including one involving 71 postmenopausal women. The women with reduced bone mineral density had lower serum vitamin K levels than those with normal bone density. Researchers also have shown that supplemental vitamin K reduces the amount of calcium lost, which indirectly benefits bones. Results of a recent study from the Netherlands showed vitamin K, when combined with calcium, magnesium, zinc, and vitamin D, substantially reduced bone loss in postmenopausal women. The daily requirement for adult women (not pregnant or nursing) is 65 micrograms. The best food sources are leafy green vegetables; kale and turnip greens provide 10 times your daily requirement. Green tea, spinach, broccoli, lettuce, and cabbage are excellent sources, but asparagus, green beans and peas, whole wheat, oats, and watercress also provide decent amounts.

Vitamin B12 also positively contributes to bone health. A recent study featured in the *Journal of Nutrition* showed that osteoporosis occurred more often in women who had marginal or deficient vitamin B12 levels. B12 is abundant in foods of animal origin—beef, clams, lamb, fish, eggs, and many cheeses. Vegans and vegetarians can be at risk for B12 deficiency and so should take a supplement or eat B12-enriched foods. The recommended daily dose of vitamin B12 for women (not pregnant or nursing) is 2 micrograms. Deficiency is rare in younger people but not unusual in the elderly.

Osteoporosis is not an inevitable part of aging. It can be prevented with proper lifestyle and diet. If caught early, it also can be treated effectively.

OSTEOPOROSIS RISK FACTORS

The National Osteoporosis Foundation has identified the following risk factors associated with osteoporosis.
- Family history, especially a parent or sibling with osteoporosis
- Early or surgically induced menopause
- Being thin with a small frame or having the eating disorder anorexia nervosa
- Abnormal menstrual periods, particularly absence of menstruation
- Use of certain medications, such as corticosteroids and anticonvulsants
- Low lifetime calcium intake
- Inactive lifestyle
- Cigarette smoking and excessive alcohol use

In addition, too much caffeine, sugar, salt, soft drinks, and animal protein also can increase your risk.

ALZHEIMER'S AND DEMENTIA

When it comes to concerns about aging, Alzheimer's disease is right up there with retirement funding. The Alzheimer's Association estimates about 4.5 million Americans have the condition. It is the most common cause of mental deterioration, or dementia, among the elderly. Dementia is medically described as a broad impairment of intellectual function that is progressive and interferes with normal social and occupational activities. Alzheimer's disease is the most common and severe form of dementia. The progressive brain degeneration of Alzheimer's disease is characterized by gradual memory loss, eventual inability to do routine tasks, disorientation, difficulty learning, eventual loss of language skills, impaired judgment, and personality changes. As the disease progresses, the person becomes increasingly unable to take care of herself as other body systems fail. Disease progression can vary dramatically.

Researchers previously suspected decreased hormonal activity, specifically estrogen production, caused cognitive decline in women. However, results of scientific studies have demonstrated just the opposite—increasing estrogen levels with HRT increases dementia rates. According to the results of a sub-study of the Women's Health Initiative (WHI), HRT doubled the likelihood of developing dementia after just one year of use. A National Institutes of Health (NIH) report evaluating the study concluded that most of the dementia cases were probably Alzheimer's. The NIH report also indicated that, based on cognitive test results in individuals not diagnosed with dementia, general brain function was negatively affected in the women given HRT.

Heavy metal toxicity, specifically aluminum, also has been linked to dementia and Alzheimer's. Aluminum in drinking water has been associated with an increased risk of the illness. The *American Journal of Epidemiology* reported results of a study in which researchers investigated the effects of aluminum and silica in drinking water. The researchers' findings support the hypothesis that drinking water with high concentrations of aluminum increase Alzheimer's disease risk. This is not conclusive proof, but it raises enough suspicion to encourage you to avoid impure drinking water and other potential sources of heavy metals.

We do not know what causes Alzheimer's, and there is presently no cure. Melvyn Werbach, MD, explains in his *Textbook of Nutritional Medicine* (Third Line Press, 1999) that 10 percent to 20 percent of dementia patients have reversible nutritional deficiencies. Werbach says poor mineral absorption or deficiencies in calcium, magnesium, iron, and zinc significantly contribute to dementia. There are several natural prevention alternatives to consider, including correcting nutritional deficiencies, normalizing homocysteine levels, and taking a few key nutritional supplements.

Folic acid and **vitamins B6** and **B12** help keep homocysteine levels in check. This toxic amino acid is a natural byproduct of bodily functions, but high homocysteine levels have been identified as a cause of heart disease. New research indicates cognitive function is negatively affected as well. Results of a study published in the *American Journal of Clinical Nutrition* showed lower concentrations of vitamin B12 and folate and higher concentrations of homocysteine are associated with poor cognitive function. Eating more green leafy vegetables or taking a dietary supplement that contains folic acid and vitamins B6 and B12 can help keep homocysteine levels in check.

Alpha-lipoic acid may be an effective antioxidant for protecting brain function, according to results of a small study published in the *Archives of Gerontology and Geriatrics*. The researchers gave nine patients with Alzheimer's disease or related dementias 600 mg of alpha-lipoic acid daily for about a year. The group treated with alpha-lipoic acid demonstrated stabilized cognitive function. Researchers concluded alpha-lipoic acid should be considered a treatment option in cases of dementia and Alzheimer's. More research is needed because this trial was not double-blind or placebo controlled. A larger test group also will provide more significant results.

Soy isoflavones also show promise as an effective preventive agent for dementia. Results of a recent study featured in *Pharmacology, Biochemistry and Behavior* demonstrated that postmenopausal women who took a supplement containing isoflavones experienced improved memory, ability to focus, and recall ability. The dose was 60 mg per day.

Ginkgo (*Ginkgo biloba*) is probably the most promising herbal treatment for Alzheimer's disease. Physicians in Germany prescribe ginkgo more than any other drug treatment for dementia. There's good reason for their confidence. In a review article published in the *Lancet*, researchers looked at more than 40 double-blind, controlled studies evaluating ginkgo's efficacy against age-related mental decline. They determined there was enough good evidence to conclude ginkgo is an effective treatment for severe age-related mental decline. In another study, published in *JAMA*, researchers gave more than 300 participants either 40 mg of ginkgo or placebo three times daily. The herbal treatment resulted in significant improvement; 27 percent of those taking ginkgo scored better on a scale that evaluates Alzheimer's disease severity compared with 14 percent in the placebo group. Further, 40 percent of those taking placebo worsened during the trial compared with only 19 percent of those taking ginkgo. Ginkgo extracts are typically standardized to contain 24 percent ginkgo flavone glycosides.

Healthful dietary choices and lifestyle habits beginning early in life are the best tools for preventing dementia and Alzheimer's disease. Research has shown that diet contributes directly to Alzheimer's disease development. Dietary fat and excess calories in old age are risk factors, but eating fish and cereal grains reduces risk. Diet contributes to Alzheimer's disease by modulating oxidative stress and inflammation. As we age, our diets should be designed to reduce free radical production and inflammation, measures that will reduce our dementia risk.

HEART DISEASE

True or false: More women die of cancer than heart disease. False, but most women believe the statement is true. The American Heart Association reports 92 percent of the women they surveyed believed heart disease was not the greatest threat to their health. Most women simply don't realize the dangers of heart disease.

According to the American Heart Association, more than one-half million women died of heart disease in 2000. More than 40 percent of all women's deaths in America are the result of heart disease, which claims the lives of nearly as many women as men. In some cases, the outlook is even worse for women. Each year, more women than men die of stroke. Women are also more likely to die within one year after a heart attack than men are. The rate of having a second heart attack is higher for women than for men. What many women don't realize is two-thirds of all women older than 50 are at risk of developing cardiovascular disease, and that heart disease causes 50 percent of deaths in women older than 50. Heart disease is most definitely a significant health concern for women.

In conventional medicine, doctors believe menopause and its associated hormonal changes are to blame for women's increased cardiovascular disease risk. However, the risk doesn't increase any faster after menopause—heart disease risk for women is a steady, straight-line increase. But conventional medical doctors think menopause is an estrogen deficiency, so they believe the lack of estrogen increases a woman's heart disease risk. Several studies, including the now-famous WHI, confirm the opposite. HRT does not protect against heart disease; it contributes to it. In fact, the American Heart Association's official position on the topic of HRT and heart disease is that HRT is not associated with any benefit in the prevention of heart disease or stroke and should not be used in postmenopausal women for the sole purpose of heart disease prevention. Because HRT also contributes to cancer and dementia, we can conclude HRT is dangerous.

HEART DISEASE RISK FACTORS

To reduce your heart disease risk, minimize, eliminate, or control as many of the following risk factors in your life as possible.
- Alcohol abuse
- Birth control pill and HRT use
- Diabetes
- Diet rich in refined carbohydrates
- Elevated cholesterol levels
- Elevated homocysteine levels
- High blood pressure
- Insufficient antioxidants, essential fatty acids, fiber, and water in diet
- Obesity
- Physical inactivity
- Smoking or being around second-hand smoke
- Stress and worry

So if decreased estrogen levels aren't causing more and more women to develop heart disease, what factors are? As you might expect, diet plays a role, as does stress. The foods to avoid should not surprise you. They include animal fat, which is rich in saturated fat; sugar and refined carbohydrates; and trans fats. The foods women may not be getting enough of to prevent heart disease include fiber- and antioxidant-rich foods. The same strategy that helps you keep your hormones in balance can help you prevent the deadly illnesses associated with aging. Dietary supplementation can also play a role in maintaining heart health.

Coenzyme Q10 (CoQ10) is a natural, fat-soluble nutrient essential for cellular energy synthesis. Heart cells require large amounts of uninterrupted energy. The average heart beats 72 times a minute or 38 million times a year. CoQ10 supports heart health by contributing to healthy circulation, blood pressure, and endurance. Researchers have found that patients with various heart conditions have CoQ10 deficiencies 50 percent to 75 percent of the time. CoQ10 has been shown to help treat various heart conditions, including angina, atherosclerosis, congestive heart failure, cardiomyopathy, high blood pressure, and mitral valve prolapse. The daily dose of CoQ10 to help prevent heart disease is 100 mg twice a day. Look for a CoQ10 product with studies proving it enters the cells; just raising blood levels may not provide the beneficial effects.

Essential fatty acids, known as beneficial fats, supply energy to the heart and promote absorption of vitamins A, D, E, and K. Essential fatty acids are not manufactured by the body and must come from food sources or supplements. Most Americans get plenty saturated fats (harmful fats) and not enough unsaturated fats (beneficial essential fatty acids). Results of population studies have revealed that those who eat diets rich in omega-3 essential fatty acids (EPA, DHA) from fish or vegetables have a significantly lower heart disease risk. Fish oils have been shown to reduce homocysteine levels (a risk factor for heart disease), maintain healthy cholesterol and blood pressure levels, support healthy circulation, and protect low-density lipoprotein (LDL) cholesterol from harmful oxidation. When considering a fish oil supplement, choose one that is derived from cold-water fish, because they are less likely to be contaminated with heavy metals and toxins. Other sources of essential fatty acids include flax and pumpkin seed oils. The recommended dose is 600 mg of an EPA and DHA blend up to three times daily or 1,000 mg flax oil capsules up to six times daily.

Folic acid and **vitamins B6** and **B12** can help reduce homocysteine levels, according to several recent studies published in the *New England Journal of Medicine* and *JAMA*. Several years ago, elevated homocysteine levels were identified as a risk factor for heart disease. Homocysteine is thought to promote atherosclerosis by damaging and weakening artery walls. Even slightly elevated levels significantly increase heart attack and stroke

UNDERSTANDING THE ESSENTIALS

Essential fatty acids (EFAs) are so called because they are critical for good health, yet the body does not produce them. You must get them from food—good outside sources are essential. Omega-3 and omega-6 fatty acids are both forms of polyunsaturated fats. Both have health benefits, but if you eat the typical Western diet, you are getting enough omega-6s and not enough omega-3s.

There are several omega-3 fatty acids, including eicosapentaenoic acid (EPA), docosahexaenoic acid (DHA), and alpha-linolenic acid (ALA). EPA and DHA are found primarily in cold-water fish, such as tuna, salmon, herring, sardines, halibut, bluefish, and mackerel. ALA is found primarily in dark green leafy vegetables, flaxseed, and certain vegetable oils. It pays to make sure you are getting your omega-3s, because researchers have found many health benefits associated with these EFAs. Omega-3s from fish oils or other sources may help improve heart health, reduce hypertension, improve rheumatoid arthritis, improve depression and other mental health symptoms, and prevent cancer.

Omega-6 fatty acids are beneficial as well, especially those with high gamma-linoleic acid (GLA) content. Good dietary sources include cereals, eggs, poultry, most vegetable oils, and whole-grain breads. There are a number of oils rich in omega-6s, including evening primrose oil, borage oil, black currant seed oil, and flaxseed oil. Omega-6 fatty acids may help reduce pain of rheumatoid arthritis; relieve discomfort of PMS, endometriosis, and fibrocystic breasts; reduce symptoms of eczema and psoriasis; improve acne and rosacea; and prevent or improve diabetic neuropathy.

Most likely you are getting plenty of omega-6 fatty acids in your diet, but do pay attention to omega-3s. Improving the ratio of these two EFAs in your diet is a worthwhile effort.

risk regardless of cholesterol levels. A diet lacking in green leafy vegetables can encourage high homocysteine levels. Supplemental B vitamins can help offset the dangerous effects of homocysteine.

Vitamins C and **E** have been identified as key nutrients for heart health. Studies featured in the *American Journal of Clinical Nutrition* and the *Lancet* concluded both of these antioxidant vitamins help prevent heart disease and reduce death rates. These antioxidants prevent free radical damage, which can harm artery walls and lead to clogs. Based on results of research, antioxidants work better in combination than they do singularly. You should get 500 mg of vitamin C three times daily and 800 IU vitamin E daily. Check your multivitamin to see if it includes beta-carotene and selenium, two other important antioxidants.

Garlic (*Allium sativum*) is a powerful antioxidant herb backed by extensive research. Several clinical studies demonstrate garlic can help prevent and even treat heart disease and the associated risk factors, including high cholesterol and high blood pressure. In one study, patients received either 800 mg standardized garlic or placebo daily for 16 weeks. Those taking garlic reduced their total cholesterol by 12 percent and triglycerides by 17 percent. In a blood pressure study involving 47 subjects, half were given 600 mg powdered garlic standardized to 1.3 percent alliin; the others received placebo for 12 weeks. The patients taking garlic lowered their systolic blood pressure by 11 percent and diastolic pressure by 13 percent.

NUMERICALLY SPEAKING

High cholesterol is a risk factor for heart disease, so it is worth explaining that the terms "good" and "bad" cholesterol are a bit misleading. Both forms of cholesterol—LDL ("bad") and HDL ("good")—are necessary. The challenge with LDL is that it is easily influenced by oxidation, which causes LDL molecules to become stickier—a risk to heart health. Both forms of cholesterol are important to many body functions. The liver uses cholesterol to manufacture hormones and bile acids for proper digestion, for example.

Maintaining the proper balance of LDL to HDL cholesterol is a more appropriate goal. Because LDL can turn into plaque, you don't want to have more than 130 mg/dl. Cholesterol levels are considered healthy when the total is less than 200 mg/dl and HDL levels are greater than 40 mg/dl.

Healthy blood pressure levels are also critical to heart health.

Normal blood pressure	120 over 80
Borderline	120–140 over 85–89
Mild	140–160 over 90–104
Moderate	160–180 over 105–114
Severe	180+ over 115+

Heart disease and its associated risk factors, such as high blood pressure, unbalanced cholesterol, and elevated homocysteine levels pose a major health threat to women. Recognizing risk factors, making appropriate dietary and lifestyle changes, and using dietary supplements will help reduce this troubling trend and allow more women to live long, vital lives.

EARLY SYMPTOMS OF HEART DISEASE

Results of a study featured in the *Journal of Cardiovascular Nursing* identified the following early symptoms of heart disease in women who had experienced a previous heart attack.
- Unusual fatigue
- Shortness of breath
- Pain in the shoulder blade/upper back

These same researchers discovered that, although women reported these symptoms, none had received a diagnosis of heart disease before their attacks.

MORE THAN SYMPTOM RELIEF

Debilitating diseases, including osteoporosis, Alzheimer's, and cardiovascular disease, are not inevitable parts of aging. We can protect ourselves from serious illnesses by getting in touch with our bodies and recognizing the underlying cause of our symptoms—imbalance.

CHAPTER 9

Reclaiming Your Healthcare

"Within my body are all the sacred places of the world, and the most profound pilgrimage I can ever make is within my own body"

—*Saraha, Buddhist saint*

To be "in our bodies" is to be able to listen to and pick up on the clues they give us. You know best the rhythms of your body and when you feel good or off. If something is bothering you, chances are you know what it might be. Don't discredit these kinds of hunches. Intuition is powerful. And remember: Mind and body are connected. There can be an innate knowing if you practice and trust this communication. By being in tune, we are better equipped to be our own healthcare advocates. By closely listening to our bodies and by finding practitioners who listen to us, we can start putting the *care* back into healthcare. As we learn to listen and care more deeply for ourselves, and as we partner with doctors who will listen and learn with us, we can live much healthier lives. If we ignore signals being sent by our bodies or if we endure with practitioners who don't spend time with us or won't really listen to what we are saying, we are putting our health in jeopardy. I know; I've seen first-hand what can happen when a woman's knowing is doubted by her healthcare provider.

I had the pleasure of working with a wonderful woman, Elaine, who was recovering from uterine cancer. She told me the most frustrating story as she choked back tears of anger, rage, and depression. Her periods were "normal," always a 28- to 30-day cycle, no pain, and a consistent moderate amount of bleeding. Around the age of 46, her periods began to get a bit irregular. She noticed in particular that her flow was getting much heavier, and she would spot between cycles. This alarmed her so she made an appointment with her general practitioner. Elaine informed me her doctor spent approximately 12 minutes with her, did a pelvic exam, said everything was fine, and dismissed her with a diagnosis of "perimenopause." Elaine tried to ask about other possibilities, such as cancer. The doctor told Elaine she was not in a risk category for cancer, so it wasn't a consideration. Well, to make a long, dreadful story short, Elaine continued to feel like something was wrong, so she continued her arduous journey of trying to be heard. After doing much research on the Internet, Elaine demanded she be referred to an OB/GYN for a more thorough exam including a biopsy. Sure enough, and to the surprise of her doctors, Elaine had advanced uterine cancer.

Unfortunately this is not an unusual occurrence. Michelle, 36, was having an array of digestive complaints and knew something was not right. She was given everything from prescription antacids to laxatives to treat her various symptoms. She was also told she was too young to have cancer, so once again it was overlooked. You guessed it. After traveling a long, frustrating road trying to get someone's attention, Michelle was diagnosed with colon cancer.

Both of these women detected an imbalance in their bodies. They knew something was wrong, but their doctors couldn't see beyond risk factors, categories, and symptom relief. When our bodies give us symptoms, they are messages. We must learn to heed these signals and find a practitioner who is willing to take time to uncover what is causing the symptom and help us address that. Finding this kind of help in healthcare isn't easy.

There is an old Buddhist saying: Every day, empty your cup. If your cup is full, there is no room for anything else. I empty my cup every time I am with a patient. This way, there is only my patient and me. My mind is not cluttered with preconceived ideas of what might be going on. I am not looking at her and ruling out this or that just because of her age, socioeconomic status, or anything else. I am open, listening, and present. My job is to meet her where she is and help her get where she is going.

For doctors not to pay attention to individuals—not to really listen—is dangerous. Doctors can use trends and risk categories as guideposts, but paying attention to what an individual is saying—actually listening with an open mind—is the key to accurately and safely partnering with someone in her health. Your doctor works for you. If you are not getting the care you believe you need and deserve, fire your doctor. I understand our current healthcare system has significantly reduced our choices through HMOs and PPOs, but we have to start somewhere with the hard work of changing the way the healthcare system and medical professionals the view patients.

Recently, a fairly famous person published a book on osteoporosis and was being interviewed on the *Today Show*. The interviewer asked the author if small-framed Caucasian women were at risk for osteoporosis, because that is what the interviewer had heard. The author responded, "I have heard that too, but I am not sure. What you need to do is ask your doctor because he is the one who knows your health history. Ask him, 'Am I at risk for osteoporosis?'" I was appalled at this advice. You should not depend on anyone else to know your health history.

It is a wise investment to collect your medical background and research your possible health risks. In addition to finding a practitioner who will listen to you, take charge of your own healthcare and become your own advocate. The following are some suggestions for doing this.

- When going to see a doctor, take a friend for support with you. This person can help you remember what was said and make sure you don't forget to ask any of your questions. (It is also a good idea to make a list of your questions so you remember to ask what is important to you.) Consider bringing a mini tape recorder to the visit to record the conversation with your doctor. This way you can revisit it later, when you are more relaxed.

- Do your homework. Make sure you gather enough trustworthy information on what might be going on with you. There is so much information available today. Go to the library; go online. You can read up on just about any set of symptoms, diagnosis, treatment, alternative treatment, prevention, and so on. Find reliable sources, even if that means consulting professionals or reading articles from medical journals. There are organizations and associations for every topic, from cancer and endometriosis to herbs and alternative practitioners.

- Know your health history and key information. Anytime anyone performs a laboratory or diagnostic test on you, request a copy. This ensures accountability and allows you to compile your own personal health history. If something arises in the future, you will be able to refer to that valuable information.

We need to reclaim power over our health, get back into our bodies, understand our own rhythms, and be able to notice if we start to get out of balance. Believe me, I understand about imbalance. I struggle each day to maintain a dynamic state of balance between my desires and responsibilities. Like anything else in life, the only way you get in balance is to swing out of it at times. I realize contrast helps us see and appreciate what is in front of us. Sometimes it takes imbalance for us to appreciate balance. Every so often you have to whoop it up, let your hair down, push the boundaries in every-thing—in eating, in love, in adventure, in all areas of life—but all with a mindfulness and an awareness of yourself and the effects of your behavior.

I also make the effort to maintain balance in my body, for my health. As I mentioned, my body sent me signals most doctors would have dismissed as perimenopause—as if this were a diagnosis at all. I knew, however, the symptoms meant I needed to pay attention to my stress levels because they affect my hormones, which affect my menstrual cycle and overall health. I also knew diet, digestion, and exercise were part of the puzzle.

What I hope you've gleaned from this book is a sense of power over your health, a sense of oneness with your body, and an understanding that, with your commitment to diet, exercise, and lifestyle, you can effect a change. By balancing your diet, finding an exercise routine for you, reducing stress, and understanding high-quality supplementation, you will improve digestion and glandular function. These improvements help correct the hormone imbalance that is causing your PMS, your "perimenopause" symp-toms, menopause symptoms, breast fibroids, or whatever "woman's complaint" you've been experiencing. The approach is multifaceted—the web has many strands—but these efforts for your overall health will not only reduce the symptoms you might be feeling today, they will reduce your risk of more life-threatening conditions later on.

The best route to health is taking good care of yourself. It is an empowering process. I urge you to take the necessary steps for yourself and for other women so we can reclaim our natural cycles of life from the medical machine.

About the Author

H olly Lucille, ND, RN, is a graduate of Southwest College of
Naturopathic Medicine in Tempe, Ariz. She received the prestigious
Daphne Blayden award for her "commitment to naturopathic medicine,
academic excellence, compassion, perseverance, a loving sense of humor,
and a positive, supportive outlook." In addition to maintaining a private
practice in Los Angeles, Calif., she is a president of the California
Association of Naturopathic Medicine and a member of Enzymatic Therapy's
scientific advisory board. Dr. Lucille has appeared on Lifetime Television for
Women and the Discovery Health Channel and has been a guest on radio
shows around the country. Holly has a sincere passion for the individual
wellness of all individuals.

Visit Dr. Lucille's web site at www.AllHealLucille.com.

Recommended Reading

Eat, Drink, and Be Healthy by Walter C. Willett, MD (Free Press, 2002)

Eat Right for Your Type by Peter J. D'Adamo, ND, and Catherine Whitney (Putnam Pub Group, 1996)

Encyclopedia of Natural Medicine by Michael Murray, ND, and Joseph Pizzorno, ND (Prima, 1998)

From Fatigued to Fantastic: A Proven Program to Regain Vibrant Health, Based on a New Scientific Study Showing Effective Treatment for Chronic Fatigue and Fibromyalgia by Jacob Teitelbaum, MD (Avery Penguin Putnam, 2001)

The Natural Pharmacist Series (Prima Publishing)

No More HRT: Menopause Treat the Cause by Karen Jensen, ND, and Lorna R. Vanderhaeghe (Quarry Health Books, 2002)

The Safe Shopper's Bible: A Consumer's Guide to Nontoxic Household Products by David Steinman and Samuel S. Epstein, MD (John Wiley & Sons, 1995)

Thyroid Power: Ten Steps to Total Health by Richard Shames, MD, and Karilee H. Shames, RN, PhD (HarperResource, 2002)

The Thyroid Solution: A Mind-Body Program for Beating Depression and Regaining Your Emotional and Physical Health by Arem Ridha, MD (Ballantine Books, 2000)

Tired of Being Tired: Rescue, Repair, Rejuvenate by Jesse Lynn Hanley, MD, and Nancy Deville (Berkley Pub Group, 2002)

What Your Doctor May Not Tell You About Menopause by John R. Lee, MD, with Virginia Hopkins (Warner Books, 1996)

What Your Doctor May Not Tell You About Premenopause By John R. Lee, MD, Jesse Hanley, MD, and Virginia L. Hopkins (Warner Books, 1999)

Women's Bodies, Women's Wisdom: Creating Physical and Emotional Health and Healing by Christiane Northrup, MD (Bantam Books, 1998)

Women's Encyclopedia of Natural Medicine by Tori Hudson, ND (Keats/NTC/Contemporary Publishing Group Inc., 1999)

References

Chapter 2

Bell MC, et al. Placebo-controlled trial of indole-3-carbinol in the treatment of CIN. *Gynecol Oncol* 2000;78:123-9.

Dwivedi C, et al. Effect of calcium glucarate on beta-glucuronidase activity and glucarate content of certain vegetables and fruits. *Biochem Med Metab Biol* 1990;43:83-92.

Garnet L. Effects of estrogen plus progestin on gynecologic cancers and associated diagnostic procedures: the Women's Health Initiative randomized trial. *JAMA* 2003;290(13):1739-48.

Heerdt AS, et al. Calcium glucarate as a chemopreventive agent in breast cancer. *Isr J Med Sci* 1995;31:101-5.

Horn-Ross PL, et al. Phytoestrogen intake and endometrial cancer risk. *J Natl Cancer Inst* 2003;95(15):1158-64.

Lamar CA, et al. Serum sex hormones and breast cancer risk factors in postmenopausal women. *Cancer Epidemiol* 2003;12:380-3.

Malejka-Giganti D, et al. Post-initiation treatment of rats with indole-3-carbinol or beta-naphthoflavone does not suppress 7, 12-dimethylbenz[a]anthracene-induced mammary gland carcinogenesis. *Cancer Lett* 2000;160(2):209-18.

Manson JE, et al. Estrogen plus progestin and the risk of coronary heart disease. *N Engl J Med* 2003;349(6):523-34.

Paolini M. On the usefulness of drug metabolizing enzyme modulation for anti-cancer strategies. *Mutat Res* 1998;405(1):113-4

Rajapakse N, et al. Combining xenoestrogens at levels below individual no-observed-effect concentrations dramatically enhances steroid hormone action. *Environ Health Perspect* 2002;110:917–21.

Walaszek Z. Chemopreventative properties of D-Glucaric acid derivatives. *Cancer Bull* 1993;45:453-7.

Walaszek Z. Potential use of D-Glucarate acid derivatives in cancer prevention. *Cancer Lett* 1990;54:1-8.

Wong GY, et al. Dose-ranging study of indole-3-carbinol for breast cancer prevention. *J Cell Biochem* 1997;28-29(Suppl):111-6.

Zanetta GM, et al. Hyperestrogenism: a relevant risk factor for the development of cancer from endometriosis. *Gynecol Oncol* 2000;79(1):18-22.

Chapter 3

Albertazzi P, et al. The effect of dietary soy supplementation on hot flushes. *Obstet Gynecol* 1998;91(1):6-11.

Allred CD, et al. Soy diets containing varying amounts of genistein stimulate growth of estrogen-dependent (MCF-7) tumors in a dose-dependent manner. *Cancer Res* 2001;61:5045-50.

Allred CD, et al. Dietary genistin stimulates growth of estrogen-dependent breast cancer tumors similar to that observed with genistein. *Carcinogenesis* 2001;22(10):1667-73.

Anderson JW, et al. Meta-analysis of the effects of soy protein intake on serum lipids. *N Engl J Med* 1995;333:276-82.

Arjmandi BH. The role of phytoestrogens in the prevention and treatment of osteoporosis in ovarian hormone deficiency. *J Am Coll Nutr* 2001;20(5):389S-402S.

Baker BP, et al. Pesticide residues in conventional, IPM-grown and organic foods: insights from the U.S. data sets. *Food Additives and Contaminants* 2002;19(5):427-46.

Branca F. Physical activity, diet and skeletal health. *Public Health Nutr* 1999;2(3A):391-6.

Center for Disease Control and Prevention (CDC). Physical activity levels among children aged 9-13 years. *MMWR Morb Mortal Wkly Rep* 2003;52(33):785-8.

Chopra M, et al. A global response to a global problem: the epidemic of overnutrition. *Bull World Health Organ* 2002;80(12):952-8.

Feigelson HS, et al. Alcohol consumption increases the risk of fatal breast cancer. *Canc Causes Cont* 2001;12(10):895-902.

Fletcher RH, Fairfield KM. Vitamins for chronic disease prevention in adults: clinical applications. *JAMA* 2002;287(23):3127-9.

Food and Drug Administration, HHS. Food labeling: trans fatty acids in nutrition labeling, nutrient content claims, and health claims. Final rule. *Fed Regist* 2003;68(133):41433-1506.

Hu FB, et al. Physical activity and risk of stroke in women. *JAMA* 2000;283(22):2961-7.

Hurley BF, Roth SM. Strength training in the elderly: effects on risk factors for age related diseases. *Sports Med* 2002;30(4):249-68.

Ilich JZ, Kersetter JE. Nutrition in bone health revisited: a story beyond calcium. *J Am Coll Nutr* 2000;19(6):715-37.

Ingram D, et al. Case-control study of phyto-estrogens and breast cancer. *Lancet* 1997;350(10):990-4.

Ivarsson T, et al. Physical exercise and vasomotor symptoms in postmenopausal women. *Maturitas* 1998;29(2):139-46.

Kiecolt-Glaser JK, McGuire L, et al. Emotions, morbidity, and mortality: new perspectives from psychoneuroimmunology. *Annu Rev Psychol* 2002;53:83-107.

Kiecolt-Glaser JK, et al. Psychoneuroimmunology: psychological influences on immune function and health. *J Consult Clin Psychol* 2002;70(3):537-47.

Kushi LH, et al. Physical activity and mortality in postmenopausal women. *JAMA* 1997;277(16):1287-92.

Liebman B. The changing American diet. *Nutrition Action Healthletter* 1999.

Moffett JK, et al. Randomised controlled trial of exercise for low back pain: clinical outcomes, costs and preferences. *BMJ* 1999;319(7205):279-83.

Morgan K. Daytime activity and risk factors for late-life insomnia. *J Sleep Res* 2003;12(3):231-8.

Okano H, et al. Effects of exercise and amenorrhea on bone and mineral density in teenage runners. *Endocrine J* 1995;42:271-6.

Oomen CM, et al. Association between trans fatty acid intake and 10-year risk of coronary heart disease in the Zutphen Elderly Study: a prospective population-based study. *Lancet* 2001;357(9258):746-51.

Salmeron J, et al. Dietary fat intake and risk of type 2 diabetes in women. *Am J Clin Nutr* 2001;73(6):1019-26.

Schreiber MD, et al. Isoflavones and postmenopausal bone heath: a viable alternative to estrogen therapy? *Menopause* 1999:6(3):233-41.

Sirtori CR. Risks and benefits of soy phytoestrogens in cardiovascular diseases, cancer, climacteric symptoms and osteoporosis. *Drug Safety* 2001;24(9):665-82.

Snow CM, et al. Serum IGF-I is higher in gymnasts than runners and predicts bone and lean mass. *Med Sci Sports Exerc* 2000;32(11):1902-7.

Van Boxtel MP, et al. Aerobic capacity and cognitive performance in a cross-sectional aging study. *Med Sci Sports Exerc* 1997;29(10):1357-65.

WHO Technical Report. Diet, nutrition and the prevention of chronic diseases. *World Health Organ Tech Rep Ser* 2003;916(i–viii):1-149.

Warren MP, Perlroth NE. Hormones and sport. The effects of intense exercise on the female reproductive system. *J Endocrinol* 2001;170:3-11.

Warren MP, Stiehl AL. Exercise and female adolescents: effects on the reproductive and skeletal systems. *J Am Med Women's Assoc* 1999;54(3):115-20.

Worthington V. Nutritional quality of organic versus conventional fruits, vegetables, and grains. *J Alt Compl Med* 2001;7(2):161-73.

Yamamoto S, et al. Soy, isoflavones, and breast cancer risk in Japan. *J Natl Cancer Inst* 2003;95(12):906-13.

Zanker CL, Swaine IL. Relation between bone turnover, oestradiol, and energy balance in women distance runners. *Br J Sports Med* 1998;32(2):167-71.

Chapter 4

Blumenthal M, et al. The Complete German Commission E Monographs—Therapeutic Guide to Herbal Medicines. Austin (TX): American Botanical Council; 1998.

Cho SY, et al. Alternation of hepatic antioxidant enzyme activities and lipid profile in streptozotocin-induced diabetic rats by supplementation of dandelion water extract. *Clin Chim Acta* 2002;317(1-2):109-17.

Coltorti M, et al. A review of the studies on the clinical use of S-adenosylmethionine (SAMe) for the symptomatic treatment of intrahepatic cholestasis. *Methods Find Exp Clin Pharmacol* 1990;12:69-78.

Ferenci P, et al. Randomized controlled trial of silymarin treatment in patients with cirrhosis of the liver. *J Hepatol* 1989;9(1):105-13.

Flora K, et al. Milk thistle (*Silybum marianum*) for the therapy of liver disease. *Am J Gastroenterol* 1998;93(2):139-43.

Fujisawa, et al. Glycyrrhizin inhibits the lytic pathway of complement—possible mechanism of its anti-inflammatory effect on liver cells in vital hepatitis. *Microbiol Immunol* 2000;44(9):799-804.

Gebhardt R. Prevention of taurolithocholate-induced hepatic bile canalicular distortions by HPLC-characterized extracts of artichoke (*Cynara scolymus*) leaves. *Planta Med* 2002;68(9):776-9.

Harmelin DL, et al. Antacid-induced phosphate depletion syndrome presenting as nephrolithiasis. *Aust N Z J Med* 1990;20(6):803-5.

Herzog P. Effect of antacids on mineral metabolism. *Z Gastroenterol* 1983;21(Suppl): 117-26.

Jarrett M, et al. Sleep disturbance influences gastrointestinal symptoms in women with irritable bowel syndrome. *Dig Dis Sci* 2000;45(5):952-9.

Kassir ZA. Endoscopic controlled trial of four drug regimens in the treatment of chronic duodenal ulceration. *Irish Med J* 1985;78:153-6.

Key TJ, et al. Body mass index, serum sex hormones, and breast cancer risk in postmenopausal women. *J Natl Cancer Inst* 2003;95(16):1218-26.

Kline RM, et al. Enteric-coated, pH-dependent peppermint oil capsules for the treatment of irritable bowel syndrome in children. *J Pediatr* 2001;138(1):125-8.

Lieber CS. Alcoholic liver disease: new insights in pathogenesis lead to new treatments. *J Hepatol* 2000;32(1 Suppl):113-28.

Locke CR 3rd, et al. Helicobacter pylori and dyspepsia: a population-based study of the organism and host. *Am J Gastroenterol* 2000;95(8):1906-13.

Logan AC, Beaulne TM. The treatment of small intestinal bacterial overgrowth with enteric-coated peppermint oil: a case report. *Altern Med Rev* 2002;7(5):410-7.

Morgan AG, et al. Comparison between cimetidine and Caved-S in the treatment of gastric ulceration and subsequent maintenance therapy. *Gut* 1982;23:545-51.

Morgan AG, et al. Maintenance therapy: a two-year comparison between Caved-S and cimetidine treatment in the prevention of symptomatic gastric ulcer. *Gut* 1985;26:599-602.

PDR for Herbal Medicines. Montvale, NJ: Medical Economics, 1998.

Safe S. Environmental estrogens: roles in male reproductive tract problems and in breast cancer. *Rev Environ Health* 2002;17(4):253-62.

Singleton DW, Kahn SA. Xenoestrogen exposure and mechanisms of endocrine disruption. *Front Biosci* 2003;8(Suppl): 110S-8S.

Starek A. Estrogens and organochlorine xenoestrogens and breast cancer risk. *Int J Occup Med Environ Health* 2003;16(2):113-24.

Verkasalo PK, et al. Circulating levels of sex hormones and their relation to risk factors for breast cancer: a cross sectional study in 1092 pre- and postmenopausal women (United Kingdom). *Cancer Causes Control* 2001;12(1):47-59.

Walaszek Z, et al. Metabolism, uptake, and excretion of a d-glucaric acid salt and its potential use in cancer prevention. *Cancer Detect and Prev* 1997;21(2):178-90.

Walker AF, et al. Artichoke leaf extract reduces symptoms of irritable bowel syndrome in a post-marketing surveillance study. *Phytother Res* 2001;15(1):58-61.

Wellington K, Jarvis B. Silymarin: a review of its clinical properties in the management of hepatic disorders. *BioDrugs* 2001;15(7):465-89.

Werbach MR. *Textbook of Nutritional Medicine.* Tarzana, Calif: Third Line Press, 1999.

Woodson GC. An interesting case of osteomalacia due to antacid use associated with stainable bone aluminum in a patient with normal renal function. *Bone* 1998;22(6):695-8.

Chapter 5

Ashok BT, et al. Abrogation of estrogen-mediated cellular and biochemical effects by indole-3-carbinol. *Nutr Cancer* 2001;41(1-2):180-7.

Chiaroni P, et al. A multivariate analysis of red blood cell membrane transports and plasma levels of L-tyrosine and L-tryptophan in depressed patients before treatment and after clinical improvement. *Neuropsychobiology* 1990;23:1-7.

Contempre B, et al. Effect of selenium supplementation in hypothyroid subjects of an iodine and selenium deficient area: the possible danger of indiscriminate supplementation of iodine-deficient subjects with selenium. *J Clin Endocrinol Metab* 1991;73:213–5.

Blumenthal M, et al. The Complete German Commission E Monographs—Therapeutic Guide to Herbal Medicines. Austin (TX): American Botanical Council; 1998.

Brody S, et al. A randomized controlled trial of high dose ascorbic acid for reduction of blood pressure, cortisol, and subjective responses to psychological stress. *Psychopharm* 2002;159(3):319-24.

Darbinyan V, et al. Rhodiola rosea in stress induced fatigue—a double blind crossover study of a standardized extract SHR-5 with a repeated low-dose regimen on the mental performance of healthy physicians during night duty. *Phytomedicine* 2000;7(5):365-71.

Eltom A, et al. Changes in iodine metabolism during late pregnancy and lactation: a longitudinal study among Sudanese women. *European J Clin Nutr* 2000;54:429-33.

Gordley LB, et al. Menstrual disorders and occupational, stress, racial factors among military personnel. *J Occup Environ Med* 2000;42(9):871-81.

Gunderson MP, et al. Effect of acute stress on plasma beta-corticosterone, estradiol-17beta and testosterone concentrations in juvenile American alligators collected from three sites within the Kissimmee-Everglades drainage basin in Florida (USA). *Comp Biochem Physiol C Toxical Pharmacol* 2003;135(3):365-74.

Hallstrom C, et al. Effect of ginseng on the performance of nurses on night duty. *Comp Med East and West* 1982;6:87-92.

Kim DH, et al. Effects of ginseng saponin administered intraperitoneally on the hypothalamo-pituitary-adrenal axis in mice. *Neurosci Lett* 2003;343(1):62-6.

Lillberg K, et al. Stressful life events and risk of breast cancer in 10,808 women: a cohort study. *Am J Epidemiol* 2003;157(5):415-23.

McAlindon TE, et al. Indole-3-carbinol in women with SLE; effect of estrogen metabolism and disease activity. *Lupus* 2001:10(11):779-83.

Need AG, et al. Vitamin D status: effects of parathyroid hormone and 1,25-dihydroxyvitamin D in postmenopausal women. *Am J Clin Nutr* 2000;71:1577-81.

Outila TA, et al. Vitamin D status affects serum parathyroid hormone concentrations during wonder in female adolescents: associations with forearm bone mineral density. *Am J Clin Nutr* 2001;74:206-10.

PDR for Herbal Medicines. Montvale, NJ: Medical Economics, 1998.

Provalova NV, et al. Mechanisms underling the effects of adaptogens on erythropoiesis. *Bull Exp Biol Med* 2002;133(5):428-32.

Shevtsov VA, et al. A randomized trial of two different doses of SHR-5 Rhodiola rosea extract versus placebo and control of capacity for mental work. *Phytomed* 2003;10(2-3):95-105.

Taylor SE, et al. Behavioral responses to stress in females: tend and befriend, not fight or flight. *Psycholog Rev* 2000;107(3):411-29.

Thilly CH, et al. The epidemiology of iodine-deficiency disorders in relation to goitrogenic factors and thyroid-stimulating-hormone regulation. *Am J Clin Nutr* 1993;57(2 Suppl):267S–70S.

Van Bakel MME, et al. Antioxidant and thyroid hormone status in selenium-deficient phenylketonuric and hyperphenylalaninem patients. *Am J Clin Nutr* 2000;72-976.

Van Cauter E, et al. Age-related changes in slow wave sleep and REM sleep and relationship with growth hormone and cortisol levels in healthy men. *JAMA* 2000;284(7):861-8.

Williams KA, et al. Evaluation of a wellness-based mindfulness stress reduction intervention: a controlled trial. *Am J Health Promot* 2001;15(6):422-32.

Werbach MR. Textbook of Nutritional Medicine. Tarzana, Calif: Third Line Press, 1999.

Wortsman J, et al. Decreased bioavailability of vitamin D in obesity. *Am J Clin Nutr* 2000;690-3.

Yoshikawa M, et al. Structures of new dammarane-type triterpene saponins from the flower buds of Panax notoginseng and hepatoprotective effects of principal ginseng saponins. *J Nat Prod* 2003;66(7):922-7.

Chapter 6

Atmaca M, et al. Fluoxetine versus Vitex agnus-castus extract in the treatment of premenstrual dysphoric disorder. *Hum Psychopharmacol* 2003;18(3):191-5.

Bhatia SC, Bhatia SK. Diagnosis and treatment of premenstrual dysphoric disorder. *Am Fam Physician* 2002;66(7):1239-48.

Blumenthal M, et al. The Complete German Commission E Monographs—Therapeutic Guide to Herbal Medicines. Austin (TX): American Botanical Council; 1998.

Borenstein JE, et al. Health and economic impact of the premenstrual syndrome. *J Reprod Med* 2003;48(7):515-24.

Broder MS, Kanouse DE, et al. The appropriateness of recommendations for hysterectomy. *Obstet Gynecol* 2000;95(2):199-205.

Health Services Research on Hysterectomy and Alternatives. Fact sheet. AHCPR Publication No. 97-R021. Agency for Health Care Policy and Research, Rockville, MD. www.ahrq.gov/research/hysterc.htm.

Hsia J, et al. Usefulness of prior hysterectomy as an independent predictor of Framingham risk score (The Women's Health Initiative). *Am J Cardiol* 2003;92(3):264-9.

Lobo RA. Menopause management for the millennium. Medscape Portals 2000.

PDR for Herbal Medicines. Montvale, NJ: Medical Economics, 1998.

Rutter CM, et al. Changes in breast density associated with initiation, discontinuation, and continuing use of hormone replacement therapy. *JAMA* 2001;285:171-6.

Squires S. Midlife without the crisis. *The Washington Post* 1999:Z20.

Thys-Jacobs S, Alvir MJ. Calcium-regulating hormones across the menstrual cycle: evidence of a secondary hyperparathyroidism in women with PMS. *J Clin Endocrinol Metab* 1995;80:2227-32.

Chapter 7

Albertazzi P, et al. The effect of dietary soy supplementation on hot flashes. *Obstet Gynecol* 1998;91:6-11.

Blumenthal M, et al. The Complete German Commission E Monographs—Therapeutic Guide to Herbal Medicines. Austin (TX): American Botanical Council; 1998.

Boerner RJ, et al. Kava-kava extract L1 150 is as effective as Opipramol and Buspirone in generalized anxiety disorder—an eight-week randomized, double-blind multi-centre clinical trial in 129 out-patients. *Phytomedicine* 2003;10(Suppl 4):38-49.

Boyle CA, et al. Caffeine consumption and fibrocystic breast disease: a case-control epidemiologic study. *JNCI* 1984;72:1015-9.

Burdette JE, et al. Black cohosh acts as a mixed competitive ligand and partial agonist of the serotonin receptor. *J Agric Food Chem* 2003;51(19):5661-70.

Christy CJ. Vitamin E in menopause. *Am J Ob Gyn* 1945;50:84-7.

Cohen AJ, Bartlik B. Ginkgo biloba for antidepressant-induced sexual dysfunction. *J Sex Marital Ther* 1998;24:139-43.

Emser W, Bartylla K. Effect of kava extract WS 1490 on sleep patterns in healthy subjects. *Neurol Psychiatr* 1991;5:636-42.

Grube B, et al. St. John's wort extract: efficacy for menopausal symptoms of psychological origin. *Advances in Ther* 1999;16(4):177-86.

Harrer G, Sommer H. Treatment of mild/moderate depressions with Hypericum. *Phytomed* 1994;1:3-8.

Hypericum Depression Trial Study Group. Effect of Hypericum perforatum (St. John's wort) in major depressive disorder: a randomized controlled trial. *JAMA* 2002 Apr 10;287(14):1807-14.

Kam IW, et al. Dietary supplement use among menopausal women attending a San

Francisco health conference. *Menopause* 2002;9:72-8.

Kohnen R, et al. The effects of valerian, propranolol, and their combination on activation, performance, and mood of healthy volunteers under social stress conditions. *Pharmacopsychiatry* 1988;21:447-8.

Laakmann G, et al. St. John's wort in mild to moderate depression: the relevance of hyperforin for the clinical efficacy. *Pharmacopsychiatry* 1998;31(Suppl. 1):54–9.

London RS, et al. Endocrine parameters and alpha-tocopherol therapy of patients with mammary dysplasia. *Cancer Res* 1981;41:3811-3.

London RS, et al. The effect of alpha-tocopherol on premenstrual symptomatology: a double-blind study. II: Endocrine correlates. *J Am Col Nutr* 1984;3:351-6.

Minton JP, et al. Clinical and biochemical studies on methylxanthine-related fibrocystic breast disease. *Surgery* 1981;90:299-304.

PDR for Herbal Medicines. Montvale, NJ: Medical Economics, 1998.

PDR for Nutritional Supplements. Montvale, NJ: Medical Economics, 1998.

Philipp M, et al. Hypericum extract versus imipramine or placebo in patients with moderate depression: randomized multicenter study of treatment for eight weeks. *BMJ* 1999;319:1534–8.

Pye JK, et al. Clinical experience of drug treatment for mastalgia. *Lancet* 1985;ii:373-7.

Schulz V, et al. *Rational phytotherapy.* New York Springer-Verlag: 1998, 78-80.

Shelton RC, et al. Effectiveness of St. John's wort is major depression: a randomized controlled trial. *JAMA* 2001 Apr 18;285(15):1978-86.

Stevinson C, et al. Hypericum for fatigue—a pilot study. *Phytomed* 1998;5(6):443–7.

Stoll W. Phytopharmacon influences atrophic vaginal epithelium. Double-blind study: cimicifuga vs. estrogenic substances. *Therapeuticum* 1987;1:23-31.

Sundaram GS, et al. Serum hormones and lipoproteins in benign breast disease. *Cancer Res* 1981;41:3814-6.

Volz HP, Laux P. Potential treatment for subthreshold and mild depression: a comparison of St. John's wort extracts and fluoxetine. *Compr Psychiatry* 2000;41(2 Suppl. 1):133–7.

Vorbach E, et al. Effectiveness and tolerance of the Hypericum extract LI 160 in comparison with imipramine: randomized double-blind study with 135 outpatients. *J Geriatr Psychiatry Neurol* 1994; 7(Suppl. 1):S19–23.

Waynberg J, Brewer S. Effects of Herbal vX on libido and sexual activity in premenopausal and postmenopausal women. *Adv Ther* 2000;17:255-62.

Werbach MR. *Textbook of Nutritional Medicine.* Tarzana, Calif: Third Line Press, 1999.

Wheatley D. Stress-induced insomnia treated with kava and valerian: Singly and in combination. *Hum Psychopharmacol* 2001 Jun;16(4):353-6.

Chapter 8

Alzheimer's Disease and Related Disorders Association. Statistics about Alzheimer's disease. www.alz.org/AboutAD/Statistics.htm. 2002.

Auborn KJ, et al. Indole-3-carbinol is a negative regulator of estrogen. *J Nutr* 2003;133(7 Suppl):2470S-5S.

Beattie JH, et al. The influence of a low boron diet and boron supplementation on bone, major mineral and sex steroid metabolism in postmenopausal women. *Br J Nutr* 1993;69:871-84.

Braam LA, et al. Vitamin K1 supplementation retards bone loss in postmenopausal women between 50 and 60 years of age. *Calcif Tissue Int* 2003;73(1):21-6.

Brandi G, et al. A new indole-3-carbinol tetrameric derivative inhibits cyclin-dependent kinase 6 expression, and induces G1 cell cycle arrest in both estrogen-dependent and estrogen-independent breast cancer cell lines. *Cancer Res* 2003;63(14):4028-36.

Devirian TA, Volpe SL. The physiological effects of dietary boron. *Crit Rev Food Sci Nutr* 2003;43(2):219-31.

Dhonukshe-Rutten RA, et al. Vitamin B12 status is associated with bone mineral content and bone mineral density in frail elderly women but not in men. *J Nutr* 2003;133(3):801-7.

Fardellone P, et al. Biochemical effects of calcium supplementation in postmenopausal women: influence of dietary calcium intake. *Am J Clin Nutr* 1998:67(6):1273-8.

Grady D, et al. Cardiovascular disease outcomes during 6.8 years of hormone therapy: Heart and Estrogen/progestin Replacement Study follow-up (HERS II). *JAMA* 2002;288(1):49-57.

Grant WB. Dietary links to Alzheimer's disease: 1999 update. *J Alzheimer's Dis* 1999;1(4,5):197-201.

Hager K, et al. Alpha-lipoic acid as a new treatment option for Alzheimer type dementia. *Arch Gerontol Geriatr* 2001;32:275-82.

Haines CJ, et al. A prospective, randomized, placebo-controlled study of the dose effect of oral estradiol on bone mineral density in postmenopausal Chinese women. *Maturitas* 2003;45(3):169-73.

Humphrey LL, et al. Postmenopausal hormone replacement therapy and the primary prevention of cardiovascular disease. *Ann Intern Med* 2002;137(4):273-84.

Iannuzzi A, et al. Dietary and circulating antioxidant vitamins in relation to carotid plaques in middle-aged women. *Am J Clin Nutr* 2002;76(3):582-7.

Jie K-SG, et al. Effects of vitamin K and oral anticoagulants on urinary calcium excretion. *Br J Haematol* 1993;83:100-4.

Joosten E, et al. Is metabolic evidence for vitamin B12 and folate deficiency more frequent in elderly patients with Alzheimer's disease? *J Gerontol A Biol Sci Med Sci* 1997;52(2):M76-9.

Kanai T, et al. Serum vitamin K level and bone mineral density in postmenopausal women. *Int J Gynecol Obstet* 1997;56:25-30.

Khaw K, et al. Relation between plasma ascorbic acid and mortality in men and women in EPIC—Norfolk prospective study: a prospective population study. *Lancet* 2001;357(9257):657-63.

Kroman N, Green A. Epidemiological studies in the Upernavic District, Greenland. *Acta Med Scand* 1980;208:401-6.

Kromhout D, et al. Inverse relation between fish oil consumption and 20-year mortality from coronary heart disease. *N Engl J Med* 1985;312:1205-9.

Liu L, Yeh YY. Inhibition of cholesterol biosynthesis by organosulfur compounds derived from garlic. *Lipids* 2000;35(2):197-203.

Mader FH. Treatment of hyperlipidaemia with garlic-powder tablets. Evidence from the German Association of General Practitioners' multicentric placebo-controlled double-blind study. *Arzneimittelforschung* 1990;40(10):1111-6.

McSweeney JC, et al. Do you know them when you see them? Women's prodromal and acute symptoms of myocardial infarction. *J Cardiovasc Nurs* 2001;15(3):26-38.

Mezquita-Raya P, et al. Relation between vitamin D insufficiency, bone density, and bone metabolism in healthy postmenopausal women. *J Bone Miner Res* 2001;16(8):1408-15.

National Osteoporosis Foundation. Disease Statistics. www.nof.org/osteoporosis/stats.htm. 2003.

Nelson HD, et al. Postmenopausal hormone replacement therapy: scientific review. *JAMA* 2002;288(7):872-81.

Nielsen FH, et al. Effect of dietary boron on mineral, estrogen, and testosterone metabolism in postmenopausal women. *FASEB J* 1987;1:394-7.

Nourhashemi F, et al. Alzheimer's disease: protective factors. *Am J Clin Nutr* 2000;71(suppl):643S-9S.

Paschalis EP, et al. Effect of hormone replacement therapy on bone quality in early postmenopausal women. *J Bone Miner Res* 2003;18(6):955-9.

Prince R. Diet and prevention of osteoporotic fractures. *N Engl J Med* 1997;323(10):701-2.

Rahman KM, et al. Indole-3-carbinol (I3C) induces apoptosis in tumorigenic but not in nontumorigenic breast epithelial cells. *Nutr Cancer* 2003;45(1):101-12.

Rapp SR, et al. Effect of estrogen plus progestin on global cognitive function in post-menopausal women: the Women's Health Initiative Memory Study: a randomized controlled trial. *JAMA* 2003 May 28;289(20):2663-72.

Riggs KM, et al. Relations of vitamin B-12, vitamin B-6, folate, and homocysteine to cognitive performance in the Normative Aging Study. *Am J Clin Nutr* 1996;63(3):306-14.

Rimm EB, et al. Folate and vitamin B6 from diet and supplements in relation to risk of coronary heart disease among women. *JAMA* 1998;279(5):359-64.

Rondeau V, et al. Relation between aluminum concentrations in drinking water and Alzheimer's disease: an 8-year follow-up study. *Am J Epidemiol* 2000;152(1):59-66.

Schaafsma A, et al. Delay of natural bone loss by higher intakes of specific minerals and vitamins. *Cri Rev Food Sci Nutr* 2001;41(4):225-49.

Schaafsma A, et al. Vitamin D3 and vitamin K1, supplementation of Dutch postmenopausal women with normal and low bone mineral densities: effects on serum 25-hydroxyvitamin D and carboxylated osteocalcin. *European J Clin Nutr* 2000;54:626-31.

Schnyder G, et al. Effect of homocysteine-lowering therapy with folic acid, vitamin B12, and vitamin B6 on clinical outcome after percutaneous coronary intervention: the Swiss Heart study: a randomized controlled trial. *JAMA* 2002;288(8):973-9.

Schnyder G, et al. Decreased rate of coronary restenosis after lowering of plasma homocysteine levels. *N Engl J Med* 2001;345(22):1593-600.

Simopoulos AP. Essential fatty acids in health and chronic disease. *Am J Clin Nutr* 1999;70(3 Suppl):560S-9S.

Steiner M, Li W. Aged garlic extract, a modulator of cardiovascular risk factors: a dose-finding study on the effects of AGE on platelet functions. *J Nutr* 2001;131(3 Suppl):980S-4S.

Tanko LB, et al. Low bone mineral density in the hip as a marker of advanced atherosclerosis in elderly women. *Calcif Tissue Int* 2003;73(1):15-20.

Van der Schouw YT, et al. Higher usual dietary intake of phytoestrogens is associated with lower aortic stiffness in postmenopausal women. *Arterioscler Thromb Vasc Biol* 2002;22(8):1316-22.

Verkasalo PK, et al. Circulating levels of sex hormones and their relation to risk factors for breast cancer: a cross-sectional study in 1092 pre- and postmenopausal women (United Kingdom). *Canc Causes Cont* 2001;12(1):47-59.

Werbach MR. *Textbook of Nutritional Medicine.* Tarzana, Calif: Third Line Press, 1999.